HOW TO

A PUPPY

A Step-by-Step Guide to Train a Happy Dog in Just 7 Days Using Positive Reinforcement. Discover the Art of Raising a Puppy to Have the Dog that You've Always Wanted

DOG TRAINING ACADEMY

This report is towards furnishing precise and reliable data concerning the point and issue secured. It was conceivable that the manufacturer was not required to do bookkeeping, legally approved, or anything else, competent administrations. If the appeal is relevant, valid, or qualified, a rehearsed person should be requested during the call.

The American Bar Association Committee and the Publishers and Associations Committee have accepted and supported this Declaration of Principles.

It is not appropriate to reproduce, copy, or distribute any portion of this report in either electronic or written methods. Recording this delivery is carefully disclaimed, and the ability of this report is not permitted until the distributor has written a license.

All rights are held. The data provided in this document is expressed honestly and predictably, like any risk, in so far as abstention or anything else, is a singular and articulate duty for the beneficiary per user to use or mistreat any approaches, procedures, or bearing contained within it. No legal responsibility or blame shall be held against the

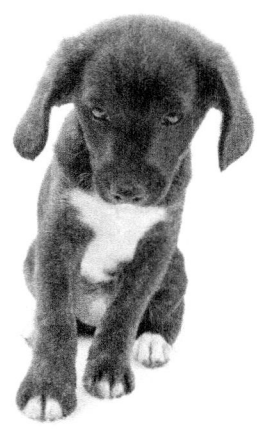

Table of Contents

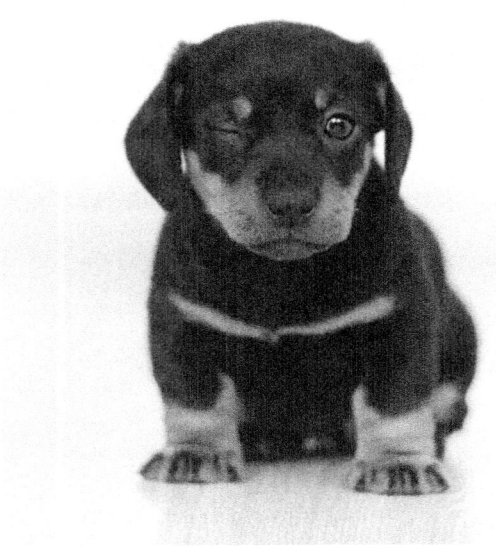

You will be training your puppy from the minute you bring it home and start instantly with the home training. Puppies begin learning from birth, and great raisers start dealing with their socialization immediately.

Some training can start when the puppy first opens its eyes and walks. Even if young doggies have limited ability to focus, they should begin at least to learn straightforward submission directions, for example, "sit," "down," and "remain," starting from as young as 7 weeks old until about 2 months old.

Formal dog training is customarily postponed until at least 6 months old. However, as a matter of fact, this adolescent stage is an insufficient time to begin. The dog is learning from each understanding, and deferring training could make it harder for the dog to learn how you might want it to act.

During the adolescent stage, the dog is starting to cement grown-up standards of conduct and gradually advances through them.

Practices learned in puppyhood may also be changed. Likewise, anything that has just been learned or trained mistakenly should be fixed and re-instructed.

Right now, we will learn how to train a puppy following a complete guide on how to train a cheerful dog in just 7 days, utilizing uplifting reinforcement.

Chapter 1.
THINGS TO KNOW BEFORE GETTING YOUR FIRST PUPPY

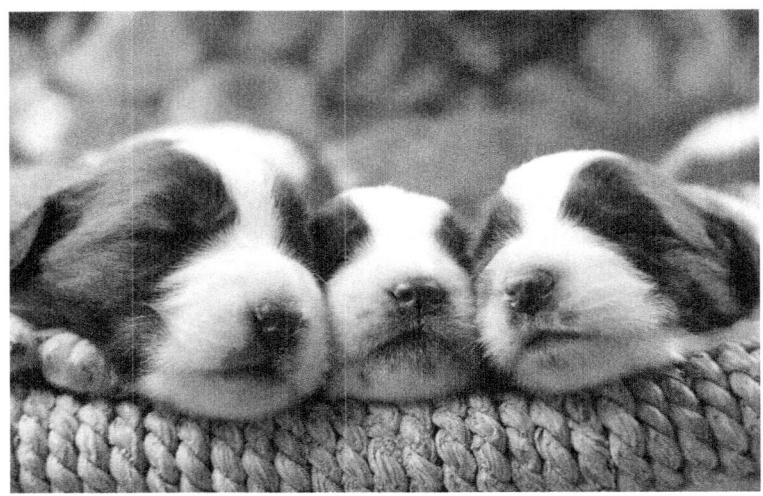

Try not to panic if your puppy seems worried: leaving her mom is a significant life change. Bringing a puppy home is very energizing for the family, but maybe not so much for the puppy, so it's your job to ensure that the transition is as smooth and optimistic as it should be.

Talk to your puppy at your discretion so that it gets used to your voice and makes an effort not to neglect it. Your puppy may initially cry in the evening, and this could be very upsetting to hear. However, you can leave lights off and attempt to abstain from letting your puppy lay down with you or your children, except if you're already set up to have a grown-up dog on your bed for the following 15 years.

Puppies are dearest sweethearts. They're small, charming, energetic, warm little creatures you can carry around all over the place. Young doggies are absolutely difficult to stand up to. Maybe this is the reason why numerous individuals wind up getting a puppy before they are trained or even before they realize how to get ready for one.

There are many choices to make and factors to consider before you decide to bring home a puppy. Try not to yield to motivation and to get home a puppy at an inappropriate time.

Do your exploration first. Learn if you are trained enough to have a puppy and discover how to get one mindfully. Get taught on the most proficient method to get ready for your new puppy and on how to raise that puppy well.

Are You for a Puppy?

Puppies might be compelling; however, they are additionally incredibly tedious sometimes. If you have never had a puppy before, at this point, you probably won't understand what you're going to get into.

Different from having a grown-up dog, raising a puppy requires a considerably elevated level of duty. Young doggies should be encouraged three to four times each day.

They should be taken outside following eating or drinking to expel properly and become house trained. Young doggies will very likely have mishaps in the home while they still learning how to be house-trained. That can mean for you a great deal of tidy up to complete.

A puppy may wake you up a few times during the night. It may be on the grounds that it needs to head outside, or it may very well be because it feels exhausted. A young puppy can't be disregarded for more than a couple of hours.

In fact, after a couple of hours, a puppy can't hold its bladder anymore (and once in a while, this applies to entrails as well). Young doggies can be a hazard and a danger if left on their own.

The puppy should remain in a box when left alone; this guides in-house training and shields the puppy from biting up everything in your home. They feel the need to investigate, bite, lick, and potentially even eat dangerous things. They don't know habits and may act boisterous or hyperactive. All doggies should be appropriately trained, and they likewise need to do a lot of activity.

These things take a great deal of time:

- Is it accurate to say that you are set up to gotten back home from work late morning to think about your puppy?
- Would you be able to deal with being woken up in the middle of the night?
- Is it safe to say that you are ready to go through a few hours of training and socialization for seven days a week, losing some of your personal free time?
- Shouldn't something be said about some other pets or individuals in your home?
- Will a puppy be excessively problematic?

If you get a young puppy, be set up to invest a ton of additional energy with it, particularly for the first hard months. In the event that this seems like excessive, yet, you, despite everything, need a dog, consider the idea of getting a grown-up dog instead.

What Sort of Puppy Is Right for You?

So, you've gauged the advantages and disadvantages of owning a puppy and concluded that all is good and well for you to bring a puppy into your family.

Congrats!

Presently it's a great time to go search for your new little buddy.

In any case, where do you start?

- First of all, decide what type of puppy is right for you. Summarize the must-have highlights or features, the ones you like, and the ones you definitely don't need.

- How enormous or little do you need your dog to be? Little dogs frequently improve better in small spaces. Nourishment, supplies, and prescriptions are progressively more costly for enormous and monster dogs than for smaller dogs.

- Do you need a dog that stays dynamic as a grown-up, or would you rather have one that will probably quiet down in a year or two? What amount of activity would you be able to give?

- Consider hair coat type too. Is it safe to say that you will manage to deal with shedding? Shedding dogs frequently need to make ordinary excursions to a groomer. Would you be able to handle the cost of this? Or, on the other hand, do you need a dog that sheds practically nothing?

- Where to locate your new puppy.

When you have gotten thought of what sort of puppy you need, it's a good time to start your hunt.

In the conceivable event, first, consider adopting a dog instead of buying it. Blended breed dogs are entirely brilliant and incredibly misjudged. Your nearby dog rescue houses or private volunteer have charming blended breed puppies simply longing for a real home.

Regardless of whether you don't know a blended breed dog could be right for you or not, your nearby Rescue Center merits a visit to meet a portion of the puppies. You may very well begin to look at them all starry-eyed!

You may genuinely have your heart set on a thoroughbred dog. Numerous individuals have a most special breed or need to know more precisely what to expect when the dog will develop. Components like the size and coat type are shocking in a thoroughbred dog.

Well-being, personality, and vitality level are details to some degree predictable, however, not ensured.

In the event that you decide to purchase a thoroughbred dog, at that point, you should be mindful. Search for an accomplished breeder with excellent notoriety. Never buy from pet stores, as their dogs regularly originate from puppy factories.

Try not to purchase a dog from a swap meet or a suspicious promotion; these young doggies have obscure origins and might be undesirable. When you locate the correct puppy for you, it will only feel right. Most dog owners will reveal to you that their dog really picked them, not the other way!

Puppy Proof Your Home

Before your little companion returns home with you, it's fundamental that you set up your home:

- Give a valiant effort to puppy evidence at each zone of your home.
- Ruinous puppy conduct is normal, disappointing, and can be dangerous for your dog if not controlled.
- Puppies can easily discover all the overlooked details that can hurt them.

Caution

Get down to a puppy eye-level and search for perils:

- Hide every single electrical line as most ideal as.
- Lock cupboards, particularly those containing nourishment or prescriptions, chemicals, harmful

synthetic compounds, and other family unit things that might be perilous.

- Keep houseplants up high where your dog can't bite their leaves.
- Get a garbage can with a cover or keep the container away from plain view.
- Keep clothing, shoes, and other little things distant. Puppies now and then bite on as well as swallow these.

The ideal approach to protect your puppy is to oversee it consistently. Keep your puppy in a closed case while you are away (simply abstain from leaving your puppy for more than a couple of hours when it is as yet young). A puppy should not have the house's full run until it is more used to and well-trained.

Stock Up on Puppy Supplies

You're going to require a lot of dog supplies before you bring home your new puppy. Start with the nuts and bolts before you end up with a lot of stuff you don't need, for example, toys your puppy loathes or beds your puppy won't stay in.

You'll certainly require a couple of fundamentals to start:

- Basic four-to six-foot rope (later you can get an extra-long one for training)
- Adjustable neckline with ID labels
- Metal or ceramic pet dishes for nourishment and water (avoid plastic as it might cause skin aggravation and is simple for puppies to bite up)
- Puppy nourishment
- Simple dog bed with space to develop
- Dog case with space to develop
- Any simple dog toys (attempt one of each: a noisy toy, a rich toy, a bite toy)
- A brush or prepping glove fitting for your puppy's coat.

As your puppy develops, you will discover you need different things, for example, training supplies and preventive items. Your vet can assist you with choosing which things best fit your dog's needs.

Locate the Right Veterinarian

Your new puppy should visit your veterinarian just before returning home with you; it is significant for the puppy to have a physical assessment, regardless of whether antibodies are expected or not. This is an opportunity to ensure there are no medical issues that went undetected by the breeder, haven, or rescue center.

It would be ideal for locating a decent veterinarian before you bring home your puppy. At that point, you will have the vet arranged and not need to hurry to discover one.

Search for a veterinary office with extraordinary notoriety in the right area for you:

- Ensure their costs are moderate for you.
- The ideal approach to locate a decent vet is to make an inquiry or two and research.
- Converse with loved ones already with pets.
- Take a gander at online audits.
- You may even need to go take a look through the medical clinic and meet the staff to learn the spot.
- On your puppy's first visit, make certain to bring all the paperwork given by the raiser or rescue center.

Your vet will do the assessment and examine the puppy inoculation plan with you. Doggies should be first vaccinated somewhere in the range of two and six months old.

Antibodies should be reinforced up until they are around 16 to 18 weeks old. You will need to visit the vet like clockwork or so up to that point.

Learn How to Raise Your Puppy Correctly

All puppies need special consideration to ensure they grow up healthy and happy.

• Choose a solid eating routine made explicitly for puppies.

• Begin house training from the minute your puppy comes home. Understand this may take numerous weeks to months.

• Begin compliance training at home; however, start little by little. Be tolerant and reliable. Nonetheless, don't be excessively severe; let your puppy be a puppy!

• Socialize your puppy well. Take your puppy loads of different places, so it can encounter sights, sounds, individuals, and pets that are new. Nonetheless, make sure just to let your puppy meet sound, inoculated dogs.

• Sign up for puppy instructional courses with a decent coach. Not only will this assist your puppy in learning, yet it will likewise encourage socialization.

• Establish a regular routine that incorporates work out.

• Stay on-plan with puppy vet visits and immunizations.

- Make time for cuddling and play. You can even show your puppy some enjoyment games.

In the event that there is more than one individual in your home who will interface with the puppy, set up the structure ahead of time.

Who is Liable for Bolstering and Strolling the Puppy and When?

Ensure all family members concur on rules about where the puppy is permitted to go. Work together to ensure the training is reliable. If there are kids in the home, ensure they realize how to behave around dogs.

In the event that there are different pets in the house, make sure they are appropriately presented and well-attended consistently.

Chapter 2.
GETTING TO KNOW YOUR DOG BEFORE TRAINING IT

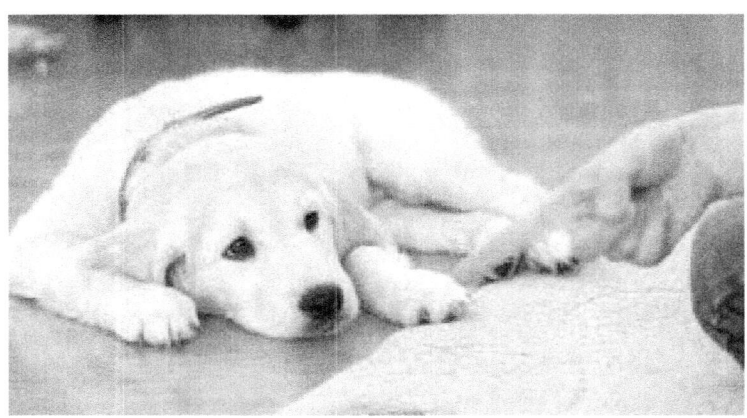

Getting to know your new puppy implies watching it and thinking about it mindfully. Carry your puppy to the vet at the earliest opportunity to discover anything you have to think about its well-being.

Also, watch its eating, restroom propensities, and physical condition. Have a go at downloading a puppy application to assist you in organizing the entirety of appropriate data.

Train your puppy, play and snuggle with it, and keep it well-trained to bond it with you and build up your figure as its pioneer and guardian.

Technique 1: Watching Health and Habit

Carry Your New Pet to the Vet

After getting your new puppy, plan a meeting with the vet. It is critical to evaluate your puppy's wellbeing, and it is an opportunity to get used to vet visits and socialization.

Ask your vet what immunizations your puppy needs and any potential medical issues you should be informed about. Keep your puppy happy and quiet, feeding it with some treats and bringing a toy along to play within the waiting room.

Monitor Your Puppy's Eating

Weaned puppies between 4 and 6 months should be fed 3 times a day to meet their health needs, while young aged doggies of half-year, or more established, should be fed only twice a day.

To build up a strong daily practice, feed your puppy on time consistently, and remove the nourishment between meals in the event that it isn't eaten.

Note the occasions when nourishment is left over, what amount is eaten, and how often your puppy asks for nourishment or appears to be ravenous. Adapt your feeding plan according to these notes if conceivable, or see a vet if your pet does not eat enough.

Track When It Goes to the Restroom

Monitoring when your puppy relaxes its bladder can enable you to foresee when it should go again and forestall future mishaps and disasters.

Also in this case, you can keep a notepad where you write down when your puppy cries to go out, or makes a mess, and you can check if there are clear examples, really connected to each other.

Attempt to bring your puppy outside, or to its assigned restroom zone (e.g., a spot on the floor covered in puppy training pads) around a similar time to those noted before, when is almost certain that your puppy needs to clear.

Keep in mind that that house training can take 4-6 months. However, it isn't unusual for mishaps to still occur with young doggies under a year old.

Get a "Puppy's Eye View" of Your Dog's Condition

To truly comprehend your puppy's everyday involvement with your home, lower yourself onto the ground at its level to watch its condition.

The rooms in your home will not be as fantastic as on your puppy's vantage point—plants overshadow it, taboo things like electrical lines and shoes are directly on its path, and some furniture is asking to be climbed onto.

Seeing things from your puppy's eyes will make its terrible conduct progressively justifiable and may assist you with revamping your house disposition in a way to be more puppy-friendly. For instance, keep wires and power outlets secured as much as could reasonably be done, and store shoes on high retires or on shoe racks where they will be less approachable.

Download a Puppy Application

There are numerous cell phone applications accessible to assist you in registering your new puppy details and progress.

These applications can help you follow your pet's weight, hypersensitivities, meds, vet arrangements, and exercise.

Likewise, you can store charming photographs, recordings, and stories about your puppy.

To assist you with finding the right application for you, here are listed a couple you can attempt:

- My Pet Diary: a free application that allows you to store your pet's data, diagram its development, arrange pictures, and record journals about it.

- Pet Minder: an application that only costs $0.99 and records significant days and occasions identified with your puppy (for example, when you began giving it a particular sort of nourishment after it last visited the vet).

Technique 2: Make a Bond with Your Dog

Give an Everyday Practice to Your Puppy

Giving an anticipated daily schedule to the puppy, for example, training, playing, and practicing it at similar times every day, is fundamental.

This helps assemble a feeling that all is well and empowers the puppy to trust in you as its owner.

Give a reasonable effort to adhere to the calendar, particularly during busy occasions, like on the memorable seasons, to enable your puppy to have a sense of security and stability.

Teach Your Puppy Its Name

Help your puppy get familiar with its name by making a positive relationship with it. Call your puppy's name and give it a treat when it reacts; in the event that it doesn't react, hurl a treat its direction each time you state its name in any case. Call your puppy's name before giving its supper or while petting it to get the puppy to begin reacting to its name rapidly.

Play with Your Puppy

All dogs react diversely to games, prodding, and roughhousing—some strongly appreciate it, while others get frightened or pestered. To test this, have a go at playing a specific game; at that point, stop, back up, and call your puppy to come to sit with you.

If it comes over cheerfully, with its head high and tail swaying, it is likely to be happy with the game; in the event that it comes through with its head and tail brought down, strolling uncertainly and not sitting when incited, it is likely discontent with the game and losing trust in you.

We recommend the following:

- Be sure to regard your puppy's breaking points and play the games it likes.
- To recover your puppy's trust, keep inciting it to come and sit, and feed it treats, and go ahead.

Train Your Puppy

Training your puppy can be a superb method to bond with it in little ordinary dosages. At around four months old, young doggies can be trained to react to fundamental directions (for example, "sit" - "remain" - "come" - "heel" - "rest") in short sessions enduring 10-15 minutes each.

Consider clicker training your puppy as a method for getting the puppy to relate the clicker with delicious treats. This will have the puppy seek you for direction and guidance and sows the seeds for potential compensation-based training.

Note: be calm around the puppy and never yell at it. Never rebuff or strike the puppy.

Keep Your Puppy Groomed

Puppies are prepped routinely by their moms during a long primary period of their lives, so they obtain the critical awareness of being thought about and cared for.

So it is likewise critical to begin prepping your new pet young with the goal that it gets used to being taken care of by its owner, groomers, and veterinarians later on. First, utilize a delicate brush and softly stroke its back, giving it a treat each couple of strokes.

If your puppy opposes, take a try at brushing it when it is sleepy and less inclined to squirm away or assault the brush.

Cuddle Your Puppy

Puppies in a litter usually snuggle together to keep warm and protect from the cold misfortune. Away from its litter, your puppy will be trying to cluster up to you, other relatives, or pets to remain warm. Enjoy your new pet and make time to nestle it, which will uplift your bond.

Guideline on Puppy Training: Reward, Tone, Positivity

Regardless of what you're attempting to show your dog, from housetraining to "heel" there are a couple of fundamental rules that will make the procedure simpler:

1. Be Reliable

Utilize a similar sign for a similar order without fail. If you use "come" multi-week, "come here" the following, and "come here, kid" the next time, you'll baffle your dog.

If your dog is permitted to pull on the rope some of the time, however, it is snapped by the neckline when it pulls on different occasions, you'll confuse it. Ensure everybody who's around your dog observes similar guidelines and utilizations similar prompts.

2. Use Applause and Prizes

Practically all advanced dog coaches retain that dogs learn better and quicker when we acclaim and prize them for hitting the nail on the head, instead of rebuffing them for failing to understand the situation. The best help is typically a blend of a little nourishment treat–particularly in the event that you train before supper time, with an exciting commendation

Try not to stress thinking that you'll end up with a dog who'll work only for nourishment.

When your dog follows what you're requesting that it does, you'll start remunerating it sporadically, and in the end, you can eliminate the treats. If your dog isn't that intrigued by nourishment, have a go at offering acclaim without the treat, or a most loved toy, or a physical prize, for example, a tremendous behind-the-ears scratch or belly rub.

3. Time the Prizes Right

The recognition and prize need to come straight following your dog have done what you need if you want it to make the right association. "Hello, at whatever point I pee outside, I get a treat. I will do this all the more regularly!"

4. Keep it Quick and Painless

Training works best if it's enjoyable and it is stopped before you both get exhausted or bored. Keep the state of mind perky, don't be like a real military instructor; make the sessions short.

Five to ten minutes is enough to begin with, or you can do numerous little instructional meetings for the day, particularly in the event that you have a very young puppy because, like children, they have shorter abilities to focus.

5. *Make it Simple for Your Dog to Hit the Nail on the Head*

When you let a dog who hasn't crapped throughout the day have a free solo run of the house, you're allowing an error that can transform into an unsolicited propensity.

When you begin rehearsing the "come" direction in a dog park, where there are a million interruptions, you're making a misstep that can transform into a negative behavior example.

Train gradually, beginning in a calm, comfortable spot without any interruptions, and step-by-step, make it even more challenging for your dog. Try not to advance to the following stage until your dog has aced the present one.

6. Keep Your Cool

Hollering, hitting, and twitching your dog around by a rope won't show it how to sit on demand, pee outside, or do whatever else you need it to do. It will instruct it that you're threatening and frightening. Good, quiet, steady training is an ideal approach to get your dog to obey and regard you.

7. Go to Class

In-person direction from a specialist coach is an ideal approach to get a well-trained dog.

Acquiescence classes are generally modest, an extraordinary method to learn how-to train, and they get your dog used to being around many different dogs and individuals. Those classes are useful for all dogs yet particularly significant for raising young doggies. To discover nearby dog mentors and styles, look at local listings.

8. Continue Rehearsing!

Try not to expect that once your dog has mastered something, it will know it and do it forever. Your dog can lose its new habits without constant ordinary practice.

Tailor Your Training to Your Dog

Each dog is extraordinary and will react better to marginally unique training styles. A few dogs are delicate to the point that a quick manner of speaking or even vivified acclaim can shake them; they need a soft, calm direction. Others are less proactive and require a lot of redundancy to become familiar with all the standards.

Furthermore, some of them will attempt to get a handle on what, precisely, your standards mean:

"Is it just right now I can't rest on the lounge chair, or anytime in all houses?"

Likewise, those dogs sometimes push back when you push them, as opposed to surrendering to what you're requesting.

Recall that albeit various dogs flourish with multiple training approaches, they all need a kind head. Hollering, hitting, and different methods that dispense agony or dread are never the answer for any dog.

They can only make a behavior issue or aggravate a current deficiency.

Training is the best thing you can do to associate and create a real bond with your dog. However, you'll have to get your work appropriately done to learn how to impart what you need and ensure that your dog will comprehend. Remain predictable and quiet; reward your dog for hitting the nail on the head and recall: you can train a dog of all ages.

Chapter 3.
TECHNIQUES AND GENERAL TIPS TO TRAIN YOUR PUPPY

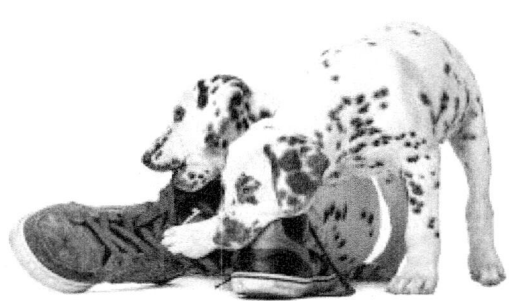

Numerous individuals can't envision existence without dogs. We respect and worship them for their dedication, unequivocal love, energetic richness, and great attitude. In any case, dogs and individuals are altogether different creatures.

Albeit formally *man's closest companions,* dogs have some natural, however annoying propensities, like bouncing up to welcome, barking, burrowing, and biting that can make it out and out hard to live with them!

To take advantage of your association with your dog, you have to show it some significant aptitudes that will help it live amicably in a human family. Learning how to train your dog will improve your life and its life, upgrade the bond among you, and guarantee its wellbeing. It also tends to be a ton of fun.

Dogs are typically anxious to learn, and the best way to progress is acceptable correspondence. Your dog needs to see how you'd like it to carry on and why it's to its own most significant advantage to conform to your desires.

Despite which strategies you use, good dog training comes down to one thing—controlling the outcomes of your dog's behavior.

If you need to impact how your dog carries on, you have to:

- Reward practices you like.
- Make certain practices you don't need or like aren't compensated.

Understand How Your Dog Learns

One of the most continuous objections of pet owners is that their dogs "just don't tune in." However, consider the situation from your dog's perspective for a minute.

If somebody was continually prattling ceaselessly in an unknown dialect that you'd never heard, to what extent would you focus?

Most likely, you wouldn't be able to focus at all.

However, this doesn't mean that you cannot communicate with your dog unless you two use the same verbal language.

To convey unmistakably and reliably with your dog, you have to observe how it learns. Dogs learn through the prompt outcomes of their conduct. Based on what these results are, they will then behave later on.

Like all other different creatures, dogs work to get beneficial things and maintain as much distance as possible from harmful things throughout everyday life.

In the event their actions bring something compensating, like nourishment, a great belly rub, recess with dog's mates, or a pleasant stroll around with its pet parent, your dog will do that conduct all the more regularly.

If an action brings about a disagreeable result like being disregarded or deprived of positive things, they find it not remunerating, and they'll do that behavior less frequently.

If You Like the Behavior, Reward It

Some training techniques use discipline, like using a choke chain or admonishing, to discourage dogs from doing everything aside from what you need them to do. Different strategies prefer not wasting time on punishments and focus on training dogs on what you do need them to do

Even if both strategies can work, the last is generally the more successful methodology, and it's additionally considerably more pleasant for you and your dog. For instance, without much of a stretch, you can use treats, games, and recognition to encourage your dog to sit down when individuals approach during strolls in the area.

If your dog is sitting, it won't be hauling you toward the individuals; it will not be bouncing up when they draw too near, it won't start mouthing on their arms and legs, etc.

That is an entirely professional training, with no agony or terrorizing required.

On the other hand, you could get your dog's rope and jolt it to the ground each time it hops up to welcome individuals, and you'd in all likelihood get a similar impact at last.

In any case, think about the conceivable aftermath:

- Your dog may conclude that individuals are frightening since it gets injured at whatever point attempts to welcome them—and may try to drive them away by snarling or barking whenever they approach.

- Your dog may conclude that YOU are alarming since you hurt it at whatever point it attempts to welcome individuals.

In the event that you can show your dog neighborly habits without harming or alarming it, why not do it?

As opposed to rebuffing it for all the things you don't need it to do, focus on teaching your dog what you do need it to do. When your dog accomplishes something you like, persuade it to do it again by compensating with something it cherishes. You'll take care of your training plans without harming the connection between you and your closest companion.

If You Don't Like the Behavior, Take Rewards Away

The most significant way of forming your dog is training that pays it to do things you like. Yet, your dog additionally needs to discover that it doesn't pay to do something you disapprove of. Luckily, discouraging undesirable behavior doesn't need to include agony or terrorizing.

You simply need to ensure those actions you hate don't get compensated. More often than not, dog inspirations aren't strange.

They just do what works! Dogs hop upon individuals, for instance, so that individuals focus on them. Therefore, they can learn not to hop up if we ignore them when they bounce up. It tends to be as necessary as just dismissing or gazing at the sky when it bounces up to welcome or play with you. Conversely, when the dog sits, you can then give it the consideration it needs.

If you adhere to this arrangement, your dog will learn two things without a moment's delay. Accomplishing something you like (sitting) will satisfy its attempts to acquire what it needs (consideration), and doing things you disapprove (hopping up) consistently brings about the loss of what it long for.

Control Consequences Effectively

As you teach your puppy dog what you do and don't need it to do, remember the accompanying rules:

- Consequences must be prompt. Dogs embrace the here and now. In contrast to us, they can't make associations among occasions and encounters that are isolated in time. For your dog to associate something it does with the outcomes of that behavior; the results must be quick. For instance, if your dog gets excessively unpleasant during play and mouths your arm, have a go at saying "OUCH!" directly; right now, you feel your teeth contact your skin. At that point, unexpectedly end recess. The message is prompt and clear: mouthing on individuals brings about not an any better time. Prizes for good conduct must come directly after that action has occurred, as well.

• The consequences must be steady. For Example, if a kid named Billy is in a study hall, responds to an instructor's inquiry effectively, finds a right pace work area, hones its pencil, and afterward punches another child in the arm in transit back to its seat. At that point, the educator says, "Great job, Billy!" and offers it a bit of sweet. What did Billy get the treatment for?

Timing is critical. So be set up to reward your dog with treats, recognition, petting, and games in the exact moment it accomplishes something you like.

• When training your dog, you—and every other person who cooperates with it—should react in a similar way to the puppy's actions each time they do them. For instance, in the event that you once in a while pet your dog when it bounces up to welcome you, while in some other cases, you holler at it instead, it will undoubtedly get confused.

How might they realize when it's alright to bounce up and when it's most certainly not?

• A few people accept that the best way to change a defiant dog into a respectful one is to overwhelm it and exercise authority over it. Nonetheless, dog training's "alpha dog" idea depends more on fantasy than on creature science. All the more significantly, it leads misinformed pet guardians to utilize training systems that aren't safe, similar to the "alpha move." Dogs who are persuasively moved onto their backs and held down can get alarmed and confounded, and they're now and again headed to bite in self-defense

Remember that dumping the "alpha dog" idea doesn't mean you need to let your dog do anything it prefers. It's OK to be the chief and make the guidelines, yet you can do that without an excessive clash.

Be a kindhearted guide, not a domineering jerk. A great chief isn't about strength and force battles. It's tied in with controlling your dog's conduct by controlling its approach to things it needs.

YOU have the opposable thumbs that open jars of dog nourishment, turn door handles, and toss tennis balls! Use them to further your best potential benefit. If your dog needs to go out, request that it sits before you open the entryway. When it needs supper, ask it to rests on acquiring it.

Do they need to take a walk?

If it's hopping up on you with enthusiasm, stand by smoothly until it sits. At that point, cut on the chain and go for your stroll. Your dog will joyfully work for all that it adores throughout everyday life. They can learn how to do what you need to procure what they need.

Training New Skills

It's anything but challenging to compensate for excellent conduct if you center on training your dog to do explicit things you like. Dogs can become familiar with a significant cluster of dutifulness abilities and engaging tricks. Choosing what you'd like your dog to learn will rely upon your inclinations and way of life.

If you need your dog to act respectfully, you can concentrate on aptitudes like "sit, down, hold up at entryways, come when called and remain." If you need to improve the quality of strolls with your dog to make them more pleasant, you can train it to walk on-leash slowly, without pulling.

Suppose you have a high-vitality dog and might want to find some activity to vent its energy. In that case, you can show it how to play, bring, play back-and-forth or take an interest in dog sports, for example, rally obedience, agility, and fly ball racing.

If you'd prefer to amaze your friends or simply invest some quality energy with your dog, you can take it to clicker training or trick instructional courses.

The conceivable outcomes are tremendous!

Training Tips

After settle which are new abilities that you'll prefer to teach to your dog, you'll be ready to begin training. To boost its learning potential and ensure you both could appreciate the training experience, remember the following fundamental tips:

- When teaching new abilities, keep instructional meetings quick and painless. Like children, dogs don't have extended capacities to focus. There's no rigid guideline, yet a perfect ordinary instructional course should not last more than 15 minutes or less. Inside that session, you can focus on one expertise or switch between a couple of various skills. To keep things engaging, have a go at doing 5 to 15 repetitions of one conduct and afterward doing 5 to 15 reiterations of another behavior. You can likewise rehearse new aptitudes and keep old ones still clear by doing a single repetition at advantageous occasions of the day. For instance, before giving your dog a delicious new bone, request that it sits or rests on acquiring it.

• Stop training while you're still ahead. End instructional meetings from a positive point of view, with the assurance your dog can progress admirably, and make sure to stop before both of you get worn out, exhausted, or disappointed.

• For dogs, English is a subsequent language. Dogs aren't brought into the world understanding it. They can get familiar with the criticalness of expressive words, as "sit", "walk" and "treat", yet when people cover those recognizable words in complex sentences, dogs some of the time experience issues comprehending. They can likewise get confounded when individuals utilize different words for something very similar. For instance, a few people will befuddle their dogs by saying, "Feathery, down!" at some point and "Plunk down, Fluffy!" one more day. At that point, they wonder why Fluffy doesn't react a similar way without fail. When showing your dog, a prompt or direction, settle on only a single word or expression, and ensure you and your family use it obviously and reliably.

• Take gradual steps with dogs, much the same as with individuals, learn best when new assignments are separated into little advances. When showing your dog another expertise, start with a simple initial step and increment difficulty level progressively. In case you're training your dog to remain, start by approaching it to stay for only 3 seconds. After some training, have a go at expanding the term of its stay to 8 seconds. When your dog has aced 8-second remain, make things somewhat harder by expanding the opportunity to 15 seconds. Throughout the following week or two, keep on bit by bit increment the length of the stay from 15 seconds to 30 seconds to a minute to a couple of minutes, and so forth. Via training deliberately and expanding trouble gradually, you'll help your dog learn over the long haul.

- Work on just a single piece of ability at a time. Many of the aptitudes we need our dogs to learn are mind-boggling. For example, in the event that you need to train a strong sit-remain skill, you'll have to deal with showing your dog that it should remain in a sitting situation until you dismiss (length); it should stay. At the same time, you move away from it (separation), and it should remain while diverting things are going on around it (interruption). You'll presumably both get baffled in the event that you attempt to show it everything of these things simultaneously. Rather, start with only one piece of the training and, when your dog has aced that, include another part. For instance, you can concentrate on the length of the exercise first. When your dog can sit-remain for a couple of moments in a tranquil spot without any interruptions while you stand directly alongside it, begin training it to remain while you move away from it. While you focus on that new part of the ability, return to approaching your dog to stay for only a couple of moments once more. When your dog can remain still while you move around the room, you can gradually develop the stay command. At that point, you can include the following part-training in all the more different conditions. Once more, when you make the ability harder by including distractions, make different parts-length and separation simpler for a brief period. In the event that you can divide and focus on all the pieces of a mind-boggling aptitude independently before putting them together, you'll set your dog up to succeed.

- If you're training your dog to explore new territory and leave the learning ground, you may have expanded the lesson's difficulty too rapidly. In the case you run into inconvenience, return a couple of steps back. Besides, if you're rehearsing a command your dog hasn't carried out for a while, and it appears to be somewhat rusty, it may require some assistance recalling what it needs to do. In the event that you run into training difficulties like these, simply revive your dog's memory by making the aptitude somewhat simpler for a couple of reiterations. Return to a stage that you realize your dog can effectively perform, and practice that for some time before attempting to increase difficulty once more.

- Practice all over, at every place. Dogs learn explicitly and don't consequently apply their insight in various circumstances and areas just as individuals do. If you show your dog to sit somewhere in your kitchen, you'll have a wonderfully kitchen-trained dog. Nonetheless, it probably won't comprehend what you mean when you request that it sits in different areas. If you need your dog to perform new aptitudes all over the places, you'll have to rehearse them in various spots; in other rooms, your yard, out on strolls, at companions' homes, at the recreation center, and anyplace else you bring your dog.

- Use real prizes to be sure to reimburse your dog with things it really finds fulfilling. A few dogs will joyfully work for dry kibbles when training in your lounge room; however, they might dislike them in case you're training in the recreation center. Since there is a more diverting condition in the recreation center, focusing is a more problematic activity for your dog. Any reward must be a prize worth working for, similar to little bits of chicken or cheddar, or an opportunity to run off-rope at the dog park with its mates. Additionally, remember that what your dog considers a prize may change at some random time. If it's already eaten a significant supper, a scratch behind the ears or a round of pull may generally be fulfilling. In the event that it hasn't eaten in some time, it'll presumably work excitedly for delectable treats.

• Being tolerant of training your dog will require some investment and exertion; however, it tends to create many good times for you both. What's more, your challenging work will pay you off. With tolerance and determination, you and your dog can achieve great goals.

An Ounce of Prevention

In the event that your puppy was over with its paws onto open electrical outlets, what might you do?

Would you sit it down and attempt to clarify for what reason that is not a smart action?

Or would you hit it on every time it repeats?

No, you'd most likely get some outlet covers. Presto! Issue understood. Prevention is, at times, the best arrangement.

When Training a dog

The most effortless approach to managing a behavior issue may be to keep the undesired action from occurring.

If your dog attacks the kitchen garbage can, you could go through weeks of training to avoid so, or you could move the junk can to a spot where your dog can't find it.

Anticipation is likewise significant in case you're attempting to train your dog to do one thing rather than another. For instance, if you need to house train your dog, it'll learn quickest if you utilize a training pad to keep it from committing errors inside while you center around teaching it to dispose of outside.

Let Your Dog Be a Dog

Numerous conduct issues can be forestalled by giving "legal", satisfactory ways for your dog to communicate its characteristic driving forces.

There are a few things that dogs simply need to do. So instead of attempting to get your dog to quit doing things like biting, mouthing, and roughhousing through and through, divert these desires the correct way.

Expanded physical movement and mental improvement are unique supplements to train.

The 7 Common Commands (Sit, Down, Stay, No, Off, Come, Heel)

Your dog is your closest companion; however, how do your relatives and neighbors feel about Fido?

For a dog to be a productive member of society, it must have great habits and comprehend an assortment of directions. Your dog ought to be confirmed, educated, inviting, and controlled.

Although dogs can learn several directions, our fuzzy companions just need to realize a couple of significant ones to exist securely around peoples and other pets.

Begin working with your dog at home on the directions beneath, and join a dog instructional course if conceivable. The lessons are fun, and they assist dogs with being amiable and dependable even with interruptions.

Moreover, be minded that all dogs need training, even those adorable little lighten balls!

Sit

This order is one of the least demanding to instruct and is generally the primary direction acquainted with a dog or puppy. Learning this order additionally enables the dog to learn how to react to train. Consider techniques that are compassionate and positive. Most significant projects use treats to inspire and remunerate dogs for fitting reactions to directions.

Down

Another functional order is down (set down). This is incredible for all dogs, yet particularly for enormous dogs. When your dog figures out how to be agreeable in a down position, you can take it with you to the recreation center or a walkway bistro. An educated dog that is loose in broad daylight is a non-risk to other pets and permits you the opportunity to appreciate a decent book or make up for lost time with companions.

Stay

Obviously, you will need to combine "remain" with sit and down. You will probably cover sit-and-down-keeps awake to a couple of moments in a puppy instructional course. However, your dog can learn how to remain for up to a half-hour or more with training. The "remain" order proves to be useful when you need your little guy to wait while you go to answer the entryway or plunk down to wrap occasion endowments.

Come

This command is essential and very important for each dog (and its owner) to achieve since it could spare their life. It is unavoidable that even with determination, your dog will one day escape through the front entryway or side door or sneak out of its rope. The "come" direction shields the dog in question from traffic, neighbors, and unpleasant experiences with other dogs.

Off

Never exchange "down" with "off." Use the "off" order to show your dog that hopping on individuals or jumping on furniture is wrong. This order is significant for training your dog to resist the urge to panic on welcome and to keep each of the four paws on the ground.

Don't Touch or No

Inquisitive dogs will discover precious objects in any place they go. Encourage them to relinquish found fortunes when you state "don't contact" or "leave it." This direction can likewise be utilized in the house if your dog discovers whatever isn't intended for dog pleasure.

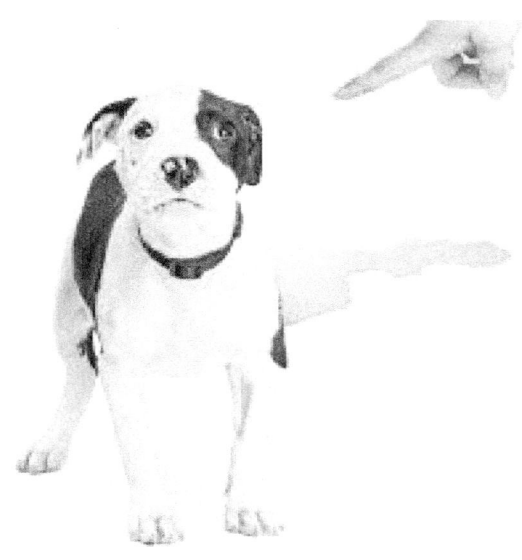

Heel or Controlled Walking

Your dog is an annoyance in the event that it pulls you down the road. Indeed, even the most extravagant dog should learn how to find a steady speed to your speed in strolling or running. There is a wide range of training methodologies you can use to show your dog to walk close by and stop and sit when you stop moving.

It's a significant feature of the capable pet owner to be able to ensure your dog comprehends essential directions. You can have a ton of fun training your dog, particularly if you discover a gathering of similar pet owners to train with.

Include bring, bounce, and different tricks to your collection, and perhaps you'll be bitten by the challenge bug. Despite your many short and long-haul objectives, start training when you are sure you can get your dog or puppy to build up great propensities at the opportune time.

Potty Training for Puppies: Choosing Your Puppy's Bathroom Location

Potty training your puppy is one of the first and most significant stages a dog owner can take to get ready for glad, sound conjunction with their pets. It's critical to do examine ahead of time and make a point to define an arrangement and calendar dependent on how much time you can commit to your dog's housetraining.

"Case" training is an indispensable piece of potty-training achievement. As nook creatures, dogs can acknowledge cases as a protected space, and as perfect animals, they'll regularly need to keep that rest space clean.

A container of the best possible size is significant, as one that is too huge may persuade the puppy, they have space to both rest and eat or dispose of. Puppy cushions give dogs the alternative of calming themselves in an affirmed spot inside.

Nonetheless, these can be precarious to train and subject to mishaps if your extreme goal is to get the little guy to just potty outside in the long run.

While house-training, perception, and supervision are fundamental, as is keeping to a timetable to make things simpler for your dog. Contingent upon the dog, potty training can also take up to several months, so tolerance is vital, as is consistency all through training.

The Most Effective Method to Train a Puppy to Pee Outside

Your puppy can't warn you when they need to ease themselves, or can they? They can in the event that you show them a "potty prompt." Potty prompts start by showing your pet the best way to flag they need to go outside. From that point, your puppy will connect the sentiment of peeing with being outside of your home. Here's the way by which to begin:

Stage 1: Teach Your Puppy the Potty Sign

Have your puppy sit by the secondary passage. When your pet barks, open the secondary passage and let them out. Or maybe you would instead not encourage your puppy to bark? Attempt a ringer. When your pet rings the chime, open the entryway and take them outside.

Keep in mind, and the potty prompt is only for going potty, don't let your puppy play a lot outside after of doing their business— else, they will connect the sign with going outside having fun, not merely going potty.

Stage 2: Determine a Set Potty Area

Put your puppy on a leash and walk them out to the piece of the yard you need your dog to alleviate themselves at. Try not to keep strolling.

Instead, trust that your pet will calm themselves. When your puppy does, reward them with treats and verbal recognition.

This will make peeing outside a positive encounter. In the event that they don't go, take your puppy back in the house and rehash. They will get on quickly.

Stage 3: Use a Crate When You're Not Home

When you aren't home with your pet, restrict them to a zone, for example, a case. This helps limit mishaps in your room, lounge room, or whatever other regions when you aren't there to hear or see the sign.

What to Do in the Event that You Have to Change the Potty Prompt

So, you trained your puppy to bark when they have to go to the restroom, yet now they bark relentlessly. You can take a stab at showing them another signal like sitting at the entryway. You could even place a floor covering by the entrance and train your puppy to realize that you open the entryway when they sit on the mat. From here, rehash stages two and three to finish your pet's retraining.

The Indoors-to-Outdoors Method

If you don't have a yard or an outdoor space where to let your dog free, it might be ideal to start potty training inside and afterward change your pet habits with the outside training.

To start training your dog to alleviate themselves in the right spot inside, you'll have to learn how to potty train a puppy on pads or how to begin with case potty training.

The Most Effective Method to Potty Train a Puppy on Pads

Decide a restricted zone to start house training—like the restroom or the pantry (in a perfect world, someplace with simple to clean floors in the event of mishaps!). Whichever area you decide on, make sure your puppy is sealed and expels any unsafe items.

Next, set up space by covering the floor with several pee pads and putting your pet's bed on a different side of the room.

To assist you in the beginning with everyday practice, here are a few stages you can follow:

Stage 1: Change pee pads frequently. However, place a little bit of the dirty cushion over the perfect pad in the zone you need your puppy to pee. The aroma reminds your puppy that this region is the toilet.

Stage 2: Remove the pee pads nearest to your pet's bed once your puppy is frequently peeing in a different zone.

Stage 3: Continue expelling the unused pee pads until you have evacuated everything except a couple of sheets.

When you have reliable accomplishment with your puppy just utilizing a couple of pee pads, you can continuously grow the zone they approach. If mishaps start to happen, diminish the territory. Pet owners who intend to progress their puppy to an indoor or yard grass "potty", relocate the pads close to this spot.

Presently, you're trained to show your puppy a potty sign so they can ease themselves outside.

Crate Potty Training

Before you start case potty training, you need the correct size control. Remember, your pet just needs enough space to stand up, pivot, and rests. Any more space will urge them to ease themselves in one corner and rest in another. You can use a few additional carton dividers so you can alter the size as they grow old.

To get your puppy used to their case, hurl a treat in and permit them to head inside and return out. Praise your puppy each time they enter. Invite your dog to stay 10 minutes in their carton and afterward once they're agreeable even for longer.

When your puppy relates their container as their living space, box potty training can start.

Rather than ruining the region where they rest and eat, they'll let you realize they have to go. Inside fifteen minutes of eating, drinking, or playing, your puppy ought to have the chance to calm down. Like other potty-training techniques, building up a routine is vital.

To What Extent Does It Take to Potty Train a Puppy?

There is no characterized time allotment with regards to how to potty train a puppy. Numerous components become an integral factor, with consistency being the most significant.

Make certain to compensate your puppy when they follow correctly their training plan.

Managing Mishaps

Mishaps will happen regardless of the amount you attempt to avoid them. It's a matter of deciding the main goal and fortifying positive conduct. Perceiving when your pet is focused or what consistently triggers mishaps will assist you with concocting restorative measures.

When tidying up messes, make sure to give the dirty territory a proper cleaning. Pet-safe stain removers and scent removers are the most suitable cleaning items to have close by.

Remember that a house-trained puppy will even have mishaps when out on the town. To restrain this behavior, keep your puppy's timetable as predictable as it could be. In case you're going out traveling or visiting companions, take your puppy on a long stroll with bunches of chances to purge their bladder sooner or later. Bringing toys is another valuable system, as they can help keep your pet concentrated on movement.

Potty training a puppy requires some investment and duty, so don't become upset. When you feel your pet is wandering out of the kilter, come back to the rudiments.

Whichever strategy you pick, stick to it and build up a daily practice. With uplifting feedback, your pet will start to perceive when they are demonstrating acceptable conduct. Make sure you're well organized by shopping for all the potty training supplies you'll require!

Housebreaking Rules for the Entire Family: Important House-Training Tips

House training your puppy is about consistency, persistence, and uplifting feedback. The main goal is to impart acceptable propensities and construct a caring bond with your pet.

As we said before, it regularly takes 4-6 months for a puppy to be completely housetrained; however, a few puppies may take as long as a year. Size can be an indicator. For example, smaller breeds have littler bladders and better capacities to burn calories and require increasingly visit outside. Your puppy's past living conditions are another indicator. You may find that you have to enable your puppy to get out from under old propensities to set up increasingly improved ones.

Besides, keeping in mind that you're training, don't stress if there are misfortunes. For whatever length of time that you proceed with an administration program that incorporates taking the puppy out at the first sign it needs to go and offering it rewards, it will learn.

When to Begin House Training Puppy

Specialists suggest that you start house training your puppy when it is between 12 weeks and 4 months old.

By then, it has enough control of its bladder and solid discharges to learn how to hold it.

In the event that your puppy is more established than 12 weeks when you bring it home and it has been dispensing within an enclosure (and potentially eating its waste), house training may take longer. You should reshape the dog's conduct - with consolation and prize.

Steps for Housetraining Your Puppy

Specialists prescribe limiting the puppy to a characterized space, regardless of whether that implies in a carton, in a room, or on a leash. As your puppy discovers that it needs to go outside to do its business, you can step-by-step give it more opportunity to meander about the house.

When You Begin to House Train, Follow These Rules:

- Keep the puppy on a customary feeding calendar and remove its nourishment between dinners.
- Take the puppy out every morning, before anything else, and afterward once at regular intervals to 60 minutes. Additionally, consistently take it outside after suppers or when it wakes from a snooze. Ensure it goes out at last around evening time, before it's forgotten.
- Take the puppy to a similar place each opportunity to do its business. Its fragrance will invite it to go.
- Stay with it outside, in any event, until it's home training.
- When your puppy manages to potty outside, acclaim it or give it a treat. A stroll around the area is a decent prize.

Utilizing a Crate to House Train Puppy

A container can be a smart thought for house training your puppy, in any event temporarily. It will permit you to watch out for it for signs on what it needs and to proceed to train it to hold it until you open the carton and let it outside.

Here are a couple of rules for utilizing a container:

- Make sure it is big enough for the puppy to stand, pivot, and rests, however not large enough for it to utilize a corner as a restroom.

- If you are utilizing the case for over two hours one after another, ensure the puppy has crisp water, ideally, in a container, you can join to the carton.

- If you can't be home during the house-training period, ensure another person offers it at all the care it needs in the day for the initial 8 months.

- Don't utilize a case if the puppy is dispensing within it. Remove it in the case of this few implications: it may have brought negative behavior patterns from the haven or pet store where it lived previously; it may not be having enough chances to go outside; the case might be too massive, or it might be too young to even think about holding it in.

Signs That Your Puppy Needs to Eliminate

Whining, crying, sniffing, barking, or, if your puppy is unconfined, barking, or scratching at the entryway, are on the whole signs it needs to go. Let it go outright.

House Training Setbacks

Mishaps are regular in puppies as long as a year old. The purposes behind mishaps go from inadequate house training to an adjustment in the puppy's condition.

When your puppy has a mishap, continue training. At that point, if it despite everything doesn't appear to be working, counsel a veterinarian to preclude a therapeutic issue.

Do's and Don'ts in Potty Training Your Puppy

Remember next do's and don'ts while housetraining your puppy:

• Punishing your puppy for having a mishap is an unmistakable no-no. It shows your puppy that it needs to fear you.

• If you get to see your puppy while it's doing right, applaud noisily so that it realizes it has finished something satisfactory. At that point, take it outside by calling it or taking it delicately by the neckline. When it's done, acclaim it or give it a little treat.

- If you found the proof yet didn't see the demonstration, don't respond indignantly by shouting or putting it to shame with it. Doggies aren't mentally equipped for associating your outrage with their mishap.

- Staying outside longer with puppy may assist with managing mishaps. It may require an additional opportunity to investigate.

- Clean up mishaps with an enzymatic chemical as opposed to a smelling salt based cleaner to limit scents that may draw the puppy back into a similar spot.

Chapter 4.

UNDERSTANDING DOG PSYCHOLOGY AND HOW THEIR MINDS WORK

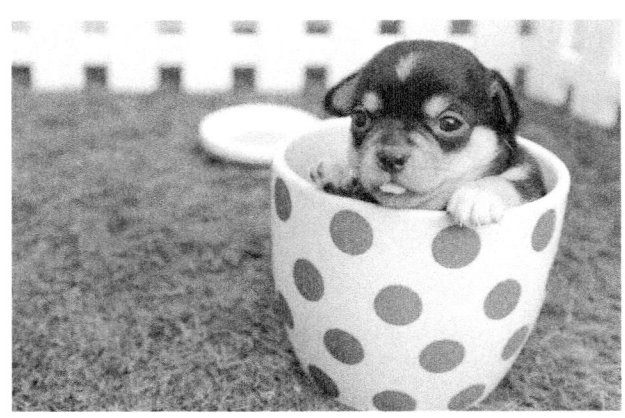

What truly goes on in a dog's brain has been an incredible subject of conversation for a long time.

What do they think?

For what reason do they think along these lines?

How could they build up this kind of thought and behavior?

While we may always be unable to directly discuss our textured mates, we have made a few stunning advances in the investigation of dog brain science that assist us with understanding them somewhat better.

Here are some of the most intriguing realities about dog brain research.

Some intriguing facts on dog brain research you most likely didn't have the foggiest idea about!

1. Dogs Can Dream

Many dog owners have presumably seen their dogs jerking, moving their paws, tenderly barking or crying, and huffing in their rest. It was generally very low considering that the dog might be able to dream, and the idea of whether a creature can really have dreamed or not was usually talked about among dog owners.

Notwithstanding, a few scientific investigations in the dog brain state with sureness that our dog companions do really encounter dreams. Dogs share comparable rest designs as people do, and their brain activity while dozing likewise takes after that of a human brain when snoozing. Because of such likenesses, it's emphatically accepted that dogs can really dream. Actually, they likely do it as much as any typical individual does. Specialists also assume that the most well-known dreams are cheerful and include exercises, such as playing, pursuing a creature, or just going around.

Some studies also show that smaller breeds will, in a general dream, more habitually than larger species and when those ongoing occasions, for example, playing, seeing an old companion, or going somewhere new, happen in real life, they can incite dreams when the dog rests.

2. They're as Smart as a Toddler

Indeed, even those without a moment of involvement with considering dog brain research realize that dogs are more brilliant than individuals who will, in general, give them kudos for. They may not be understanding complex math conditions, yet they're typically not effectively tricked, and they learn rapidly. Precisely how brilliant do they generally get in contrast with people?

Research shows that numerous dogs have insight and comprehension keeping pace with a human baby of around two years of age. They can learn how to check, comprehend around 150 words, and tackle issues just as creating tricks to play on individuals and different creatures.

3. They Understand Vocal Tones

While their jargon may never arrive at the multifaceted nature of even a small kid, our comprehension of dog brain science shows that they can understand a wide scope of vocal tones without much of a stretch.

For instance, your dog may comprehend their name and respond when called; however, according to the manner of speaking or the tone of voice used when calling, the dogs can change their behavior when they come to you.

Glad tones make a dog energized and lively, while irate tones cause dogs to feel miserable or terrified. If there is dread in your voice, the dog may accept that you're being compromised and hurry to secure you. Sharp tones of agony may incite the dog to have rescue conduct.

4. There's Something Else Entirely to Tail-Wagging than Meets the Eye

One of the most fundamental and acknowledged bits of dog brain science is presented through the trademark tail swing sign. It's broadly acknowledged by everybody from individuals who have never claimed to be experts in dog brain research that a swaying tail implies that a dog is cheerful, yet it's a more muddled subject than you may suspect.

The facts demonstrate that when a dog is cheerful, they say it with their tail. In any case, this is possibly not obvious when the tail is being swayed to one side.

In fact, if the tail is swaying to one side, it's characteristic of dread. Low tail sways mean apprehension, and fast tail sways blended in with tense muscles can be an indication of aggression.

5. Dogs Experience Jealousy

Another typically known reality about dog brain science is that dogs have felt similarly as individuals do. They clearly experience real feelings like joy, dread, and misery, yet shouldn't something be said about progressively confused sentiments, for example, envy?

Studies confirm that dogs show indications of feeling jealousy. Not precisely the same way as people experience it; however, despite everything, they give indications of managing the green-look at the beast.

Analysts put dogs one next to the other and gave them directions. The two dogs would play out a similar given order, and just one would get a treat. The dog that was not offered a treat demonstrated hints of disturbance: avoided contact with the remunerated dog and scratched all the more regularly.

This was also attributed to a desire factor, as these indications showed up more as often in investigations with sets of dogs than when one was separated from the other and did not receive any prize.

An intriguing part of their envy feeling is in the absence of signs of importance on what is offered as a prize. In the event that one dog receives something extraordinary as a treat, for example, a bit of steak, while another gets something like a little dog scone, the indications of envy are absent. They just consider that they get compensated, not what the price is.

6. No Guilt in a Dog's Eyes

It's a commonplace scene for each pet owner to enter into a room and find something that is been ruined by their dog. It's additionally a recognizable scene to detect your favorite fuzzy companion sitting, close to the zone affected, with a very tragic appearance and wet eyes. It's anything but difficult to accept this is the dog communicating regret for their activities, yet that is not, in fact, the real situation. When a dog sees the appearance of dissatisfaction on their owner's face or hears outrage and disillusionment in their voice, they respond contrarily with looks of pity.

It's also conceivable that they understand there will be negative ramifications for their activities and become tragic due to it. It's, even more, a circumstance for lamenting getting captured and not because they feel remorseful for doing something very terrible.

Strangely, dogs respond similarly regardless of whether they played out the disaster themselves or not.

As it's improbable that one dog could effectively point out another dog for wrongdoing, the dog is aware that there are the conditions of being in an unlucky spot. Simply observing or hearing the antagonism from their owners or envisioning discipline they will deserve is sufficient to produce that dismal puppy dog's face.

7. Dogs Learn from Dog Mentors

Numerous individuals go to dogs' brain science books and advisers to help them in training their dogs. Nonetheless, the nearness of a trained, more experienced dog might be the most straightforward approach to show them how to carry on and respond to directions.

Doggies usually model their conduct from more advanced dogs in their family. If the more established dog is trained well and carries on, the puppy can rapidly receive the dog's conduct.

When the more experienced dog is given a direction, performs it, and gets a treat, the puppy might have the option to understand more effectively what an order implies and what to do when it is given through a type of command.

8. No Need for Revenge

A few times in a dog owner's life, they could swear that their dogs are acting severely as an approach to seek revenge for something.

For example, a dog making a mess on the rug while its owners are gone throughout the day, or throwing a cushion since its owners would not like to play outside can, without much of a stretch be seen as vindictive acts. Nonetheless, these practices can undoubtedly be clarified through other more probable reasons.

For instance, the primary dog could have gone to the restroom on the rug since it was worried about being home alone throughout the day or having an exceptional change in schedule. The second dog could have been disappointed by repressed vitality from not being played with and discharged that vitality by destroying something.

The significant issue with the possibility of revenge in a dog is that it requires some type of intention that dogs don't appear to have. Dogs can counter-react instantly, for example, when they're assaulted, yet they don't seem to have the psychological ability to design out and perform demonstrations of retaliation against anybody intentionally.

Keep in mind that even in this case, these terrible demonstrations should always be treated through appropriate techniques, not with discipline.

9. Dog's Thrive on Love and Discipline

While giving your dog a lot of adoration and consideration is a significant part of raising an upbeat dog, studies in dog's brain science express that this by itself isn't adequate enough to raise a genuinely and intellectually reliable dog.

Dogs need a sound equalization of friendship, consideration, and control to have a sense of safety, protection, happiness, and to feel like a genuine piece of the family.

In the event that they don't get some type of control through viable and steady training and their owners taking a dominant position, they can, without much of a stretch, become troubled, impulsive, and shaky, befuddled in what is and isn't proper behavior.

Chapter 5.

CURES FOR KINDS OF BEHAVIOR ISSUES

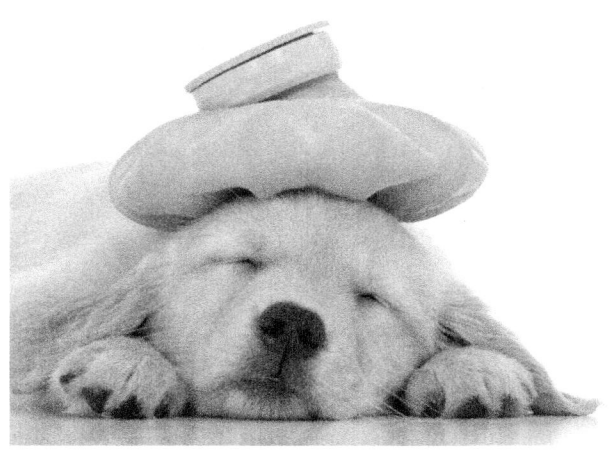

When the behavior of dogs is unfortunate, there are three different possible options:

1) Behaviors are inside the typical range for the species, age, and breed. In these cases, the owners need direction on the best way to adequately deal with the practices.

2) Some behaviors become progressively troublesome or testing. Since they may fall inside or just past the scope of what is viewed as ordinary, they are especially hard to oversee. These behaviors are things like mouthing, pee control, mounting, barking,

pursuing, predation, or overactivity. Nonetheless, this is what could be typical for the breed, however unsatisfactory for the family and home. These cases require a continuous direction and appraisal of the actions.

3) Behaviors that are irregular or pathologic because of psychological well-being issues.

These may have been created because of genetic elements, distressing prenatal condition (pre-birth, neonatal), lacking early socialization, ailments influencing brain wellbeing and advancement, or some especially awful natural occasions. The treatment of these pets, for the most part, requires behavior alteration, regularly in blend with medicine (common items, diet, and drugs) to improve fundamental pathology and encourage learning.

For most dogs to overcome these mental issues, advising from veterinary staff or mentors and quality assets are required, likewise as an active direction from a coach.

Coaches should be chosen depending on their qualifications and carefully evaluated to guarantee they use support-based training systems. Punishment–based systems should not be utilized in training. In a best-case scenario, they serve just to stifle unfortunate behavior and can prompt dread, shirking, and even hostility.

Some examples of these mental issues are, for instance, improper play (e.g., nipping or grunting at individuals); wild actions (e.g., pulling, thrusting, bouncing up, mounting, over-activity), and a few types of barking, dangerous practices, and house dirtying.

Suppose the issue is discovered to be irregular behavior. In that case, goals will require a mix of conduct adjustment methods and drugs to help restore a progressively normal mental state and encourage new learning.

Social Behavior of Dogs

The dog's social structure has been alluded to as a pack progression; however, this doesn't wholly or precisely portray the relationship of dogs with different dogs or with individuals.

Logical examinations into the behavior of wild wolves have set up that the wolf pack is really a nuclear family, with the grown-up guardians managing the herd's exercises. The dog likely has an origin from the dim wolf 12,000–14,000 years prior, even though some of the inceptions of training may reach outback 30,000 yr.

Correspondence and connections are set up through a language of visual signs, such as body stances, outward appearances, tail and ear posture, piloerection, vocalization, fragrances, and pheromones.

In any case, reproducing, taming, and contact with human beings have generated broad differences from wolf to dog, as well as among breeds, morphology, breed attributes, disposition, behavior issues, variety in social neoteny, and social flagging.

Truth be told, Huskies hold a large portion of the social flagging collection of wolves, German Shepherds around ⅔, and Cavalier King Charles Spaniels only a very little. In this way, it might be hard for dogs (and individuals) to peruse and decipher the signs of different dogs, particularly those of various mixed breeds. Early socialization, for a wide assortment of dogs, is a significant element of intraspecific correspondence.

The term strength doesn't depict the connection between two individuals; it is a relative term set up by estimating the asset to everyone and the aggregate impacts of learning.

The pecking order in dogs is neither static nor direct because the inspiration to acquire and hold a particular asset, together with past learning, characterizes the connection between two individuals for each experience.

Steadiness is kept up by reverence and not by agonistic practices.

Just in those connections in which one individual reliably concedes to another across assets and collaborations, a direct various leveled connection between the individuals may be depicted.

Even though these definitions apply to the intraspecific correspondence and contact between individuals from an animal group (e.g., dog-dog), it doesn't "decipher" the correspondence between species (e.g., dogs-people).

Associations with individuals are not built up by predominant/accommodating social flagging; they are an aftereffect of hereditary qualities and socialization and formed by learning and outcomes.

Actually, dogs have obtained a capacity and training to react to human behavior not found in wolves, regardless of whether the little wolf cub is raised in captivity.

Therefore, dog owners need to learn to examine the visual signaling and vocalization of the dog to understand when they need to attract and when they don't, just like training and rewarding good behavior and changing scary and strong practices safely and appropriately.

Chapter 6.
COMMON DOG BEHAVIOR ISSUES

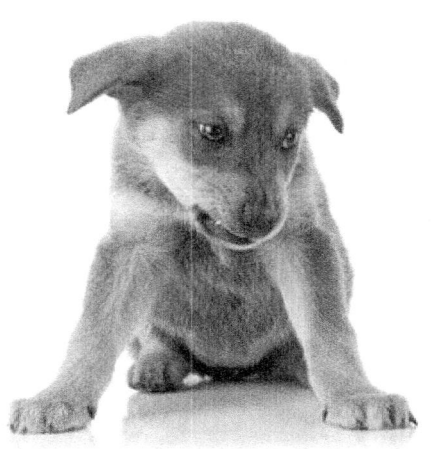

Aggression

Aggression is the most well-known and most genuine conduct issue in dogs. It's additionally the primary motivation behind why pet owners look for professional assistance from behaviorists, mentors, and veterinarians.

What Is Aggression?

The expression "aggression" alludes to a wide assortment of practices that happen for a huge number of reasons in different conditions.

Every single wild creature is forceful when guarding their domains, safeguarding their posterity, and ensuring safety for themselves for all intents and purposes.

Species that live in groups, including both individuals and dogs, use hostility and the danger of aggression to keep harmony and arrange social communications.

To state that a dog is "aggressive" can mean an entire host of things. Hostility incorporates a scope of practice that typically starts with alerts and can finish in an assault. Dogs may prematurely end their endeavors anytime during a forceful experience.

A dog that demonstrates hostility to individuals, for the most part, displays some piece of the following progressively extreme practices:

- Becoming exceptionally still and unbending
- Guttural bark that sounds compromising
- Lunging forward or accusing the individual, without contact
- Mouthing, just as to move or control the individual, without applying huge weight
- "Muzzle punch" (the dog truly punches the individual with its nose)
- Growl

- Showing teeth
- Snarl (a blend of snarling and going on the defensive)
- Snap
- Quick nip that leaves no imprint
- Quick nibbling that tears the skin
- Bite with enough strain to cause a wound
- Bite that causes cut injuries
- Repeated nibbling in fast progression
- Shake and bite

Dogs don't generally follow this succession, and they regularly do a few of the practices above all the while. Commonly, pet owners don't perceive the admonition signs before a bite, so they see their dogs as unexpectedly going off the wall crazy. Notwithstanding, that is once in a while the case. It very well may be only milliseconds between a notice and a nibble; however, it is true that dogs may occasionally bite without giving some kind of caution in advance.

Classification of Aggressive Behavior

If your dog has been forceful before you speculate that it could get aggressive, set some effort to assess the circumstances that have disturbed it to the point of generating this negative reaction.

Who endured the worst part of its hostility? When and where did it occur?

What else was going on at that point?

What had simply occurred or was going to happen to your dog? What appeared to stop its aggression?

Finding out the responses to these inquiries can explain the conditions that trigger your dog's forceful response and give knowledge into the motivations for its conduct. You need a precise conclusion before you can efficiently support your dog.

Forceful conduct issues in dogs can be characterized in various ways. A valuable way to understand why your dog is forceful is to understand the capacity or reason for the aggression.

If you consider aggression along these lines, you can learn what rouses your dog to act forcefully and recognize what it would like to obtain from its inappropriate behavior.

Territorial Aggression

A few dogs will assault and bite a gatecrasher, regardless of whether the "intruder" is a companion or adversary. Dogs' wild family members are territorial. They live in a specific region, and they protect this region from gatecrashers.

Wolves are even more profoundly territorial. If a coyote or a wolf that's not part of a pack attacks their region, the occupant wolves will assault and drive off the intruder. A few dogs show similar inclinations. They bark and charge at individuals or different creatures infringing on their home turf.

Dogs are regularly esteemed for this degree of territorial behavior. Nonetheless, as we said, a few dogs will assault and bite a gatecrasher, regardless of whether the intruder is a companion or enemy, and this could be an issue. Territorial hostility can happen along within limits routinely watched by a dog or at the boundaries of its owner's property.

Different dogs show territorial hostility just toward people or other individuals coming into the home. Male and female dogs are similarly inclined to territorial hostility. Young doggies are occasionally territorial too. This conduct typically shows up as young pups develop into pre-adulthood or adulthood, from one to three years old.

Defensive Aggression

Dogs may show forceful behavior when they imagine that one of their relatives or companions is at risk. Dogs are social animal species. In the event that they were left individually, they would still live respectively in little gatherings, or herds, of loved ones.

If one individual from a herd is in harm's way, the others regularly surge in to help protect it. This is a delegated defensive hostility, in light of the fact that the dogs are securing one of their own. Pet dogs may show a similar kind of forceful conduct when they imagine that one of their relatives or companions (human or creature) is in hazard.

In some cases, dogs reserve defensive hostility for people they consider mostly helpless. A dog who has never demonstrated hostility to outsiders in the past may begin acting forcefully when they have a litter of puppies. Similarly, a dog may initially show defensive hostility when its owner carries a little human into the family.

While this conduct sounds engaging from the start, issues emerge when the defensive dog begins to treat everybody outside the family, including companions and family members, as dangers to the child's security. Both male and female dogs are similarly inclined to defensive hostility. Young doggies are infrequently defensive. Like territorial conduct, defensive aggression generally shows up as puppies develop into pre-adulthood or adulthood, from one to three years old.

Possessive Aggression

Numerous dogs demonstrate the inclination to protect their assets from others, regardless of whether they have to or not. Dogs descend from wild predecessors who needed to seek nourishment, now settle and mates locally to endure.

Even though our pet dog will never again face such unforgiving real factors, many, despite everything, tend to protect their assets from others naturally. A few dogs' possessive inclinations are only regarding their nourishment.

These dogs may respond forcefully when an individual or another creature draws close to their nourishment bowl or approaches them while they're eating. Different dogs protect their bite bones, their toys, or things they've taken.

Still, others watch their most loved resting places, their cartons, or their beds (Often, these dogs additionally monitor their owners' beds!).

Less common are dogs who guard their water bowls. Typically, a possessive dog is anything but difficult to distinguish because they're just forceful when they have something they desire.

In any case, a few dogs will conceal their treasured things around the house and guard them against clueless individuals or creatures that have no clue that they're attempting to get almost an esteemed article.

Male and female dogs are similarly inclined to possessive hostility, and this kind of aggression is very common in both puppies and grown-ups.

Fear of Aggression

A frightened dog may get forceful whenever cornered or caught. When creatures and individuals fear something, they like to escape from that thing. This is known as the flight reaction. In any case, if getting away from a dangerous situation isn't a choice, most creatures will change to a battle reaction. They attempt to protect themselves from alarming things.

Therefore, a dog can fear an individual or another creature. At the same time, it will assault if it thinks this is the only plan of action. A fearful dog will regularly embrace frightful stances and retreat; however, they may get aggressive whenever cornered or caught.

A few dogs will grovel at the fear of being physically attacked but then assault when an undermining individual goes before them. Fearful dogs now and again flee from an individual or creature that startles them; however, if the individual or animal goes to leave, they come up from behind and nip. This is the reason it's a smart thought to abstain from walking out close to a fearful dog. The hostility due to dread is identified by fast nips or bites because a frightened dog is roused to nibble and afterward flee. Now and again, the hate doesn't start with clear warnings. A fearful dog probably won't go on the defensive or snarl to caution the unfortunate casualty off.

In this circumstance, the main admonition is the dog's fearful stance that endeavors to withdraw. Male and female dogs are similarly inclined to fear aggression, and this kind of hostility is regular in both young and grown-up dogs.

Protective Aggression

Persuaded by a dread, protectively aggressive dogs conclude that the best resistance is a decent offense. Firmly identified with aggression due to fear is protective hostility.

The essential distinction is the methodology used by the dog. Protectively forceful dogs are as yet roused by dread; however, they conclude that the best defense is always the offense rather than attempting to withdraw.

Dogs who are protectively aggressive display a blend of frightened and hostile stances. They may at first aim at an individual or another dog who terrifies them, barking and snarling. Whether or not the unfortunate casualty freezes or advances, the protectively forceful dog regularly conveys the primary strike.

Just if the unfortunate casualty withdraws, then the protectively aggressive dog is prone to end an assault prematurely. Male and female dogs are similarly inclined to guarded hostility.

It's somewhat more typical in grown-ups than in puppies, essentially because dogs need to have some self-confidence to utilize this protective methodology, and young doggies are generally less sure than grown-ups.

Sex-Related Aggression

Unsterilized male dogs will, in any case, strive for consideration of females in heat, and females will even go after a male. Although companion dogs occasionally have the opportunity to reproduce, unsterilized male dogs will try harder to get the female.

Unsterilized male dogs some of the time challenge and battle with other male dogs in any event, even when no females are available. Battling can likewise generate between dogs living respectively in a similar family. In the wild, this is versatile because the most experienced dogs are bound to pull in females for reproducing first.

In a similar manner, females living respectively in a similar family unit may contend to set up which female gains admittance to a male for reproducing. This kind of hostility is uncommon. It's watched regularly in reproductively flawless dogs and less frequently in virgin females. In the event that sex-related aggression occurs, the dogs included are for the most part at any rate from one to three years old.

Can Aggression Be Cured?

Owners of aggressive dogs regularly ask whether they can ever be certain that their dog is "restored."

Taking into account the behavior adjustment procedures that influence aggression, our present comprehension is that the instance and recurrence of certain kinds of hostility can be diminished and occasionally dispensed with.

In any case, there's no assurance that a hostile dog can be restored. Most of the time, the main arrangement is to deal with the issue by constraining a dog's presentation to the circumstances, individuals, or things that trigger its aggression.

There's consistently a hazard when managing a forceful dog. Pet guardians are liable for their dogs' actions and should avoid potential risks to guarantee that nobody's hurt.

Regardless of whether a dog has been polite for quite a long time, it's impractical to anticipate when all the fundamental conditions may meet up to make "the ideal tempest" that triggers its aggression.

Dogs that have a past filled with aggression episodes used as a method for managing distressing circumstances, can depend on that technique. Pet guardians of hostile dogs should be reasonable and need to consistently expect that their dog isn't relieved or stopped from the simple will of not letting down their owner.

Barking

Barking is one of the numerous types of vocal correspondence for dogs. Dog owners are regularly satisfied that their dog barks since it cautions them the intrusion of unwanted individuals to their home or it lets them know there's something that the dog needs.

Nonetheless, sometimes a dog's barking can be extreme. Since barking it is used for various assortments of reasons, you should distinguish its motivation and your dog's needs for barking, before you can treat the issue.

Each sort of barking may indicate a different request, and if the pet guardian manages it and train it properly, the dog will learn how to utilize it to its advantage.

For instance, dogs who effectively bark for consideration proceed to bark for different things, similar to nourishment, play, and strolls. Hence, it's imperative to train your dog to hush upon signal in a way to stop its "seek attention" related barking and instruct it to do another conduct instead—like sit or down—to get what it needs.

Numerous owners can recognize why their dog is barking just by hearing the particular bark.

For example, a dog's bark sounds distinctive when it needs to play if contrasted with how it barks when it needs to roll in from the yard. If you need to lessen your dog's barking, it's critical to understand why it's doing it.

It will require investing some time to train your dog to bark less. Lamentably, it's simply not practical to find a convenient solution or to expect that your dog will quit barking inside and out. (Would you anticipate that an individual could ever quit talking through and through?)

Your objective ought to be to diminish, instead of a wipeout, the measure of barking. Remember that a few dogs are more inclined than others. Likewise, a few breeds are known as "barkers", and it tends to be more diligently to diminish barking in dogs of these breeds.

Why Do Dogs Bark?

Territorial Barking

Dogs can bark exorbitantly because of individuals, dogs, different creatures inside their homes or moving toward their domains. Your dog's territory incorporates the region encompassing its house and, in the end, anyplace it has investigated or relates unequivocally with you: your vehicle, the course you go for during strolls, and different spots where it invests a great deal of energy.

Alert Barking

If your dog barks at any and every noise and sight, paying no much heed to the unique situation, it's likely alert/caution barking. Dogs using alert barking, as a rule, have stiffer non-verbal communication than dogs barking to welcome, and they frequently move or jump forward an inch or two with each bark.

Caution barking is different from territorial barking in that a dog may use alert barking at sights or sounds in any area whatsoever, not precisely when it's safeguarding natural territories, for example, your home, yard, or vehicle.

Attention Seeking Barking

A few dogs bark at individuals or different creatures to request consideration or prizes, similar to nourishment, toys, or play.

Greeting Barking

Your dog may be barking in welcome if it barks when it encounters individuals or different dogs, and its body is loose, it's energized, and its tail is swaying. Dogs who bark when welcome individuals or different creatures may also whimper for the emotion.

Compulsive Barking

A few dogs bark unnecessarily in a tedious manner, mind-numbingly repetitive. These dogs frequently move monotonously also. For instance, a dog who's habitually barking may run to and from along the fence in its yard or pace up and down in its home.

Socially Facilitated Barking

A few dogs bark exorbitantly just when they hear different dogs barking. This sort of barking happens in the social setting influenced by other dogs in the area.

Frustration Induced Barking

A few dogs bark exorbitantly just when they're set in a disappointing circumstance, similar to when they can't get to mates or when they're limited or tied up with all their movements confined.

Different Problems That Can Cause Barking

Ailment or Injury

Dogs at times bark in light of agony or an agonizing condition. Before endeavoring to determine your dog's barking issue, if you don't mind, you should have your dog inspected by a veterinarian to preclude therapeutic causes.

Detachment Anxiety Barking

Unnecessary barking because of separation uneasiness happens just when a dog's guardian is gone or when the dog is disregarded. For the most part, you'll observe at any rate one other partition uneasiness side effect too, such as pacing, the breaking of something, mishaps, or different indications of pain. For more data about this issue, see the section, Separation Anxiety, on the following pages if it's not too much trouble.

What to Do About Your Dog's Excessive Barking

The initial move toward diminishing your dog's barking is to decode the sort of bark your dog is communicating with. The following questions can push you to precisely settle on which kind of barking your dog is doing, so you can best address this concern. Consider your responses to these inquiries as you read through the data beneath the various kinds of barking and their remedies.

1.   When and where does the barking happen?
2.   Who or what is the objective of the barking?
3.   What things (objects, sounds, creatures, or individuals) trigger the barking?
4.   For what reason is your dog barking?

If It's Territorial Barking or Alarm Barking

Territorial behavior is frequently propelled by both dread and expectation of apparent risk. Since safeguarding an area is such a high need to them, numerous dogs are profoundly energetic to bark when they identify obscure individuals or creatures close to commonplace spots, similar to their homes and yards.

This significant kind of inspiration implies that when barking, your dog may overlook rebuffing reactions from you, for example, reproving or hollering.

Regardless of whether the barking itself is smothered by discipline or not, your dog's inspiration to guard its region will stay stable, and it may endeavor to control its domain in another manner, for example, gnawing abruptly. Dogs take part in territorial barking to alarm others to guests' nearness or frighten away gatecrashers or both. A dog may bark when it sees or hears individuals going to the entryway, for example, the postal worker carrying the mail and the upkeep individual perusing the gas meter.

It may likewise respond to the sights and hints of individuals and dogs passing by your home or condo. Also, a few dogs get particularly disturbed when they're in the vehicle and see individuals or dogs cruise by.

You should have the option to make a decision from your dog's body stance and assess whether it's barking to state "Welcome, enter!" or "Hello, you would be wise to take off. You're not welcome at my place!"

In case you're managing a dog in the last classification which isn't inviting to individuals, you'll be increasingly useful in the event that you limit your dog's capacity to see or hear bystanders and instruct it to connect the nearness of outsiders with beneficial things, for example, nourishment and consideration.

For territorial barking treatment, your dog's inspiration ought to be decreased just as its chances to safeguard its region. To deal with your dog's behavior, you'll have to obstruct its capacity to see individuals and creatures.

Removable plastic film or shower-based glass coatings can help darken your dog's perspective on territories that it watches and monitors from inside your home. Utilize secure, murky fencing to surround outside regions your dog approaches.

Try not to permit your dog to welcome individuals at the front entryway, at your front yard door, or your property limit line. Instead, train it to go to another area, similar to a carton or a tangle, and stay calm until it's welcome to welcome fittingly.

Alert barking is fundamentally the same as territorial barking in that sight, and sounds activate it. In any case, dogs who bark to alert may do so in light of things that frighten or upset them when they're not on recognizable turf.

For instance, a dog who barks territorially because of seeing outsiders moving toward will typically possibly do so when in its own home, yard, or vehicle.

Conversely, a dog that routinely cautions barks may snarl when it sees or hears outsiders drawing nearer in different spots, as well. Although territorial barking and alert barking are somewhat different, the proposals underneath them apply to the two issues.

"Calm" Training

In the event that your dog keeps on disturbing or territorially bark, despite your endeavors to hinder its introduction to sights and sounds that may trigger its barking, attempt the accompanying methods:

- Teach your dog that when somebody goes to the entryway or passes by your property, it's allowed to bark until you state "Calm." Allow your dog to bark three to multiple times. At that point, say "Calm." Avoid yelling. Simply state the direction obviously and serenely. At that instant, go to your dog, tenderly hold its jaw shut with your hand and rehash "Calm." Release your dog's jaw step away and summon it from the entryway or window. At that moment, request that your dog sits and give it a treat. In the event that it remains adjacent to you and stays calm, keep on giving it visit treats for the following couple of moments until whatever set off its barking is gone. If your dog resumes barking immediately, rehash the arrangement above. Do likewise outside if it barks at bystanders when it's in the yard.

- If you instead not hold your dog's jaw or if doing so appears to alarm your dog or make it a battle, you can attempt an alternate strategy. When your dog barks, approach it, tranquility state "Calm", and afterward brief its quietness by giving it a constant flow of modest, pea-sized treats, for example, chicken, wieners orbits of cheddar. After enough reiterations of this arrangement, possibly more than a few days or a much greater amount of training, your dog will start to understand what "Calm" means. You'll realize that it's getting it if it reliably quits barking when it hears you state "Calm." At this point, you can steadily extend the time between the sign, "Calm", and your dog's prize. For instance, say "Calm", hold up for 2 seconds, and afterward, feed your dog a few little treats in succession. Over numerous repetitions, slowly increment the time from 2 seconds to 5, and then 10, and then 20, etc.

- If the "Calm" strategy is ineffectual after 10 to 20 endeavors, at that point permit your dog to bark to multiple times, serenely state "Calm", and afterward promptly make a surprising clamor by shaking a lot of keys or an empty soft drink can load up with pennies. In the event that your dog is adequately alarmed by the sound, it'll quit barking. The moment it does, summon it from the entryway or window, request that it sits, and gives it a treat. If it remains adjacent to you and stays calm, keep on giving it treats for the following couple of minutes until whatever set off its barking is gone. In the event that it continues barking immediately, rehash all the steps.

- If your dog barks at individuals or different dogs during strolls, occupy it with unique treats, similar to chicken, cheddar, or wieners before it starts to bark. (Delicate, scrumptious treats work best.) Show your dog the treats by holding them before its nose, and urge it to snack at them while it's strolling past an individual or dog that might ordinarily make it bark. A few dogs do best if you request that they sit as individuals or dogs pass. Different dogs like to continue moving. Ensure your acclaim and prize your dog with treats whenever it decides not to bark.

• It may assist with having your dog wear a head strap now and again when it's probably going to bark (for instance, on strolls or in your home). A strap can have a diverting or quieting impact and make your dog more opposed to bark. Ensure you reward it for not barking. (Significant note: For wellbeing reasons, possibly let your dog wear the bridle when you can direct it.)

• If your dog frequently barks territorially in your yard, keep it in the house during the day and oversee it when it's in the yard with the goal to observe if it barks merely its head off when nobody's near. If it's ready to start an unnecessary alert barking (when you're not there with it, for instance), that conduct will get more grounded and harder to lessen.

- If your dog regularly barks territorially in your vehicle, instruct it to travel in a case while in the car. Traveling in a case will confine your dog's view and diminish its inspiration to bark. In the event that crating your dog in your vehicle isn't practical, attempt to have your dog wear a head bridle in the car. (Significant note: for security reasons, possibly let your dog wear the strap when you can regulate it).

Anti-Bark Collars

There is an assortment of gadgets intended to train dogs to diminish barking. Frequently, these are collars that convey an unsavory feeling when your dog barks. The upgrade may be a boisterous commotion, an ultrasonic clamor, a shower of citronella fog, or a concise electric stun.

The collars that convey commotion are inadequate with most dogs. One investigation found that the citronella neckline was at any rate as compelling for taking out barking as also the electronic neckline, and this was seen all the more emphatically by owners.

Essentially, all dogs become "neckline shrewd", implying that they learn not to bark while wearing their bark suppressant; however, they return to barking when they're not wearing them. Collars that work on a mouthpiece framework to get the sound of a dog's bark ought not to be utilized in a multi-dog home in light of the fact that any other dog barks can activate the neckline.

Hostile to bark collars are discipline gadgets and are not suggested as a first decision for managing a barking issue. This is particularly valid for barking that is propelled by dread, nervousness, or impulse.

Destructive Chewing

It's typical for young doggies and dogs to bite on objects as they investigate the world. Biting achieves various things for a dog. For young dogs, it's a method to calm the agony that may be brought from the release of new teeth.

For more established dogs, it's a method for keeping jaws stable and teeth clean. Biting likewise battles fatigue and can mitigate mellow tension or dissatisfaction.

Rule Out Problems That Can Cause Destructive Chewing

Separation Anxiety

When the dog is left alone: the animal long for ways out to meet the owner and can destroy doors, windows, blinds, etc., and get seriously hurt. As mentioned in the previous chapters, it does not do it as revenge but as a consequence of a state of uncontrolled anxiety.

In addition, they show different indications of serious nervousness, e.g., whining, barking, passing, anxiety, peeing, and pooping. There are problems related to separation in which the animal does not seem to experience a state of anxiety, but rather frustration or boredom—no need to confuse causes.

Texture Sucking

A few dogs lick, suck and gnaw at textures. A few specialists believe that this conduct comes about because of having been weaned too soon (before seven-week or two months old). In the event that a dog's texture-sucking behavior happens for protracted timeframes and it's hard to divert it when it endeavors to stop it, it's conceivable that the issue needs urgent intervention.

Hunger

A dog on a calorie-limited eating regimen may bite to protest, trying to discover extra wellsprings of nourishment. Dogs usually direct this sort of biting toward objects identified with nourishment or things that smell like nourishment.

How to Reduce or Manage Your Dog's Destructive Chewing

Puppy Teething

The longing to examine fascinating articles, and the inconvenience of getting new teeth out, could propel young doggies to bite. Like human babies, young pups experience a phase when they lose their infant teeth and experience torment as their grown-up teeth come out. This strengthened biting stage, for the most part, finishes by a half-year-old.

Some suggest giving young doggies ice 3D squares, unique dog toys that can be solidified or solid wet washcloths to bite, which may help numb getting teeth torment. Although doggies do need to bite on things, your delicate direction can show your puppy to limit biting to relevant articles, similar to its own toys, instead of biting everything around them.

Normal Chewing Behavior

Biting is very typical conduct for dogs, on equal terms. In fact, both wild and pet dogs could go through hours biting bones. As we said earlier, this movement keeps their jaws stable and their teeth clean. Dogs love to bite on bones, sticks, and pretty much whatever else accessible.

They even bite for entertainment only, or they bite for incitement, and they bite to diminish tension. While biting conduct is typical, dogs direct their biting conduct toward improper things off and on.

Both puppies and grown-up dogs must have an assortment of fitting and appealing bite toys. In any case, only giving the correct things to bite isn't sufficient to forestall bad biting habits. Dogs need to realize what is alright to bite and what isn't. They should be instructed in a delicate, accommodating way.

Helpful Tips

• "Dog-evidence" your home. Set significant articles aside until you're sure that your dog's biting behavior is confined to fitting things. Keep shoes and garments in a shut nearest, filthy clothing in a hamper, and books on racks. Make it simple for your dog to succeed.

• Provide your dog with its very own lot of toys and unpalatable bite bones. Focus on the sorts of toys that keep biting for significant stretches of time and keep on offering them. It's optimal to present something new or rotate your dog's bite toys each couple of days, so it doesn't get exhausted with the regular old toys. (Important advice: Only give your dog common bones that are sold explicitly for biting. Try not to give it cooked bones, similar to the remaining T-bones or chicken wings, as these can fragment and genuinely harm your dog. Additionally, remember that some extreme chewers might have the option to chip little pieces off of normal bones or chip their own teeth while biting. If you have worries about what's safe to give your dog, talk with its veterinarian.)

• Offer your dog some palatable things to bite, similar to menace sticks, pig ears, rawhide bones, pigskin rolls, or other common bites. Dogs can sometimes choke on eatable bites, particularly if they gnaw off and swallow enormous chunks. If your dog is inclined to do this, ensure it is isolated from different dogs when it bites so it can unwind. (This because If it needs to bite within sight of other dogs, it may feel that it needs to contend with them and attempt to swallow down eatable things rapidly.). Also, make sure to watch out for your dog at whatever point it takes a wrong shot at a consumable bite, so you can mediate if it begins to choke.

• Identify times of the day when your dog is on the way to bite and give it a riddle toy loaded up with something tasty. You can incorporate a portion of your dog's day-by-day apportion of nourishment in the toy.

• Discourage biting unseemly things by showering them with biting obstacles. When you first utilize an obstruction, apply a limited quantity of a bit tissue or cotton fleece. Tenderly spot it straightforwardly in your dog's mouth. Permit it to taste it and afterward let it out. In the event that your dog finds the taste undesirable, it may shake its head, slobber, or regurgitate. It will not fancy getting the bit of tissue or fleece once more. At this point, it will have taken in the association between the taste and the scent of the obstruction, and it'll be bound to abstain from biting things that smell like it. Use the same method on all articles that you don't need your dog to bite. Reapply the obstruction consistently for two weeks to about a month. It would be ideal if you understood, notwithstanding, that fruitful treatment for ruinous biting will require something more than just the utilization of obstructions. Dogs need to realize also what they can bite just as what they can't bite.

• Do your best to administer your dog during every waking hour until you feel certain that its biting conduct is leveled out. In the event that you see it licking or biting a thing, it shouldn't, state "Oh goodness", remove the item from your dog's mouth, and replace it with something that it CAN bite.

• When you can't oversee your dog, you should learn how to keep it from biting on wrong things in your absence. For instance, if you work during the day, you can leave your dog at home in a restricted region for as long as six hours. Utilize a box or put your dog in a little stay with the entryway or a child door shut. Make sure to remove everything that your dog shouldn't bite from its restriction territory, and give it an assortment of suitable toys and bitable things to appreciate. Remember that in the event that you restrict your dog, you'll have to provide it with a lot of activities and quality time with you when it's not limited.

• Provide your dog with many physical exercises (recess with you and with different dogs) and mental incitement (training, social visits, and so forth.). In the event that you need to disregard your dog for more than a brief timeframe, ensure it has been out for a decent play session already.

• To help your dog get familiar with the distinction between things it can bite and things it shouldn't bite, it's critical to abstain from befuddling it by offering undesirable family things, similar to old shoes, socks, etc.

It isn't reasonable to think that your dog should be aware that a few shoes are alright to bite and others aren't.

- Some puppies and adolescent dogs like to bite messy clothing. This issue is quickly settled by continually placing messy clothing in a shut hamper instead of leaving them around. Similarly, a few puppies and dogs like to assault the trash and bite up disposed napkins and tampons. This can be exceptionally dangerous. Dispose of napkins and tampons in a compartment that is out of reach of your dog.

What Not to Do

- Try not to show your dog the harm it did and beat, admonish, or rebuff it sometime later. It can't associate your discipline with some conduct; it did hours or even minutes prior.
- Try not to utilize conduit tape to hold your dog's mouth shut around a bit item for any period of time. This is coldhearted, will show your dog nothing, and dogs have passed on because of this system.
- Try not to attach a harmful article to your dog. This is unfeeling and will show your dog nothing.
- Try not to leave your dog in a container for long timeframes (over six hours) to forestall biting.
- Try not to muzzle your dog to forestall chewing.

Mounting and Masturbation

Mounting, pushing (humping) and masturbation are typical practices displayed by most dogs. Dogs jerk off in different manners. They mount and push against different creatures, individuals, and items, for example, wadded-up covers, dog beds, and toys. Once in a while, dogs simply rub against individuals or articles (without mounting them), or they lick themselves.

Puppies frequently mount and mound their littermates, different companions, individuals, and toys. A few specialists accept that this conduct works as training for future sexual experiences.

As doggies arrive at sexual development, they begin to mount different dogs in sexual settings. After they're grown up, numerous male and female dogs proceed to mount and even jerk off in light of the fact that they have discovered that the activity makes them feel better.

Sterilized dogs will regularly stroke off whenever kept from moving toward a female in heat. Frequently, during romance, females in heat mount their male "suitors." Female dogs additionally regularly mount and mound different females when one or both are in heat.

Sexual Behavior

Masturbation is a piece of typical sexual behavior for both experienced and virgin dogs. Both male and female dogs mount different dogs, individuals, and items. Many people don't understand that this action isn't restricted to only male dogs, nor do they realize that experienced dogs can show erections and discharge simply like virgin ones.

Explicitly propelled mounting and masturbation are frequently joined by "coy" non-verbal communication and romance conduct (tail up, ears pivoted in reverse, licking, pawing, play bows, and so forth.).

Play Behavior

Sexual behaviors, including mounting and pushing, are also a piece of typical play conduct. Dogs don't usually show erections or discharge with regards to play. Some dogs unnecessarily mount different dogs in light of play requesting. They don't appear to realize how to play well and get overstimulated during the game.

Reaction to Stress or Excitement

A few dogs react to unpleasant or energizing circumstances by mounting or stroking off. For example, after meeting another dog or individual, a stirred and energized dog may mount another dog, its owner, or a close-by object, similar to a dog bed or a toy.

Compulsive Disorders

Jerking off can turn into an enthusiastic propensity, particularly if a dog does it in light of pressure. Impulses like mounting and jerking off can meddle with a dog's typical activity.

Social Behavior

Dogs, now and then, mount different creatures and individuals to show well-being or control. A dog mounting thus might show an erection, yet it's probably not going to discharge.

Medical Problems to Rule Out

Different medical issues, including urinary tract diseases, urinary incontinence, priapism (tireless, regularly excruciating erections), and skin hypersensitivities, can impact a dog's mounting conduct. These issues can be very serious if not appropriately treated and require restorative consideration instead of a conduct treatment.

Dogs are experiencing one of these or other medical issues frequently invest a great deal of energy licking and biting the genital territory. If you notice your dog too much mounting, licking or biting himself, or scouring its body against things, take it to a veterinarian to preclude medical concerns.

What to Do About Excessive Masturbation and Mounting

In the event that you figure your dog may get forceful if you prevent it from mounting different dogs, individuals, or articles, don't endeavor to do as such.

Instead, counsel a certified proficient, for example, a Certified Applied Animal Behaviorist (CAAB or Associate CAAB) or a board-confirmed veterinary behaviorist (Dip ACVB). In the event that you can't locate a behaviorist in your general vicinity, you can look for help from a Certified Professional.

If you instead counsel a Dog Trainer (CPDT), then make sure to find out if they have professional training and broad experience effectively treating hostility, as this sort of skill isn't required for CPDT confirmation.

Chapter 7.
TOP TECHNIQUES TO TRAIN YOUR DOG

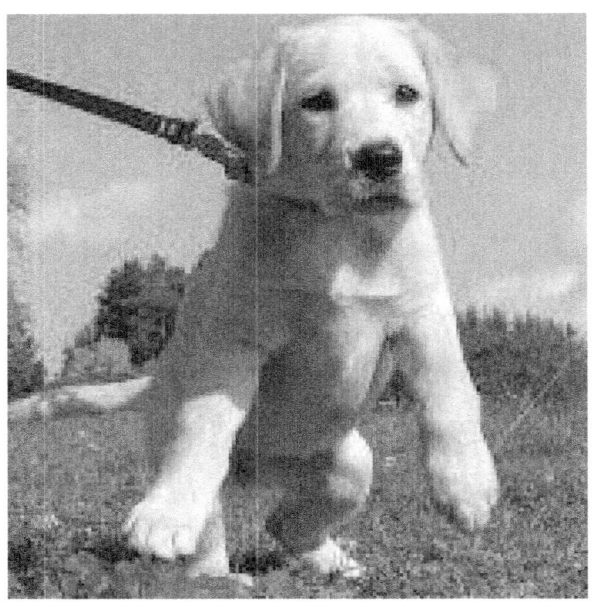

Train Your Dog to Use Its Paws

The trick of a dog giving you its paw is a basic yet exceptionally engaging one. It won't take long for you to train your dog to do it; however, it should just be educated in short blasts over a couple of days. In the long run, your dog will have the option to give you its paw and afterward even shake paw-to-hand with you.

Most dogs will do about anything to satisfy their owners. Dogs are commonly anxious to get applause and fondness, which is why training is done in the right way and can create a great outcome in a brief period. For instance, you can train your dog to shake your hand rapidly and effectively. Despite the fact that this specific direction isn't one for compliance, it is adorable and fun. A few people will show their dog how to shake their hands while others favor a progressive direction of "Give me five, Paw", "Put it there", and so forth.

Notwithstanding, relatives and companions will be intrigued by the trick your dog can perform. At that point, when it had aced the shake direction, you could proceed onward to others and even more propelled tricks. Right now, I will give you instances of how you can train your dog to shake rapidly and effectively:

- Start by picking the direction word or expression that will be utilized and afterward be steady, as it is fundamental not to confuse your dog.
- Next, you can train your dog to shake using the left or right paw or both.
- Make sure you have a couple of little yet delicious treats in your pocket, which will be utilized as a prize, alongside verbal commendation and petting.

- Tapping your dog's paw from underneath, urge it to lift its paw while giving it the picked direction.

- Hold its paw for around five seconds, trailed by a treat and applause.

- Repeat the lifting and holding steps, holding up a couple of moments longer before lifting the paw, and afterward, consistently give a prize commendation when the paw is in your grasp.

- With training, your dog will before long comprehend that when you state the order word, it is to lift the paw with or without a treat, albeit uplifting feedback as recognition and petting should be given unfailingly.

- To train your dog to shake, experience five instructional sessions each day until it finally gets it.

- If you are keen on showing your dog to shake with the other paw or the two paws, essentially experience the procedure utilizing the ideal paw or rotating with the two paws for every session.

After the "sit" command, the shake trick is one of the most effortless for a dog to learn. Usually, you can have your dog shaking in about a week or less. Truth be told, with somewhat more time and exertion, you can show your dog to play out the trick essentially by pointing at the paw.

How to Show Your Puppy to Wave?

After acing 'Shake Hands' 'Shake' command, you can instruct how to 'Wave' to your puppy. Ask your dog to 'shake hands' direction to your dog, reach down to take its paw, yet don't contact the paw.

Haul your hand back merely out of paw reach and state, "Great Wave" its paw is noticeable all around, hanging tight for you to take it. The majority of the dogs attempt to arrive at your hand and put their paw noticeable all around.

Be cautious with this direction in light of the fact that your puppy will be confounded on the grounds that you give the order and you didn't take the paw as you should.

Praise your dog merrily while your dog's paw is noticeable worldwide, so they realize this is the correct move for the direction.

After rehearsing 20 - multiple times, your dog will understand that when you state 'shake hands wave', you won't take the paw.

Quit saying 'Shake hands' and simply request that your dog 'wave' presently. If the dog just lifts a paw, however, it doesn't wave; give the directions in progressively lively mode.

Reach for your dog's paw to urge it to stretch out its paw to you and move it. Make sure to keep these instructional meetings short.

The High Five

This trick expands upon the last one of showing your dog to give you the paw. If you have not trained your dog to provide you with the paw, at that point, it is ideal for instructing that trick before endeavoring this one.

You were making sure of always having a few treats good to go. Grasp a treat and afterward lift your hand somewhat higher than you did in the past trick. The purpose behind this is to get your dog to believe that you are doing the paw trick. The dog will, at that point, raise its paw towards yours.

When your dog does this, say the order 'High Five' at that point, reward the dog in question with the treat. In the event that you have the paw trick aced with your dog, at that point, you will locate this one simple, and it won't take long for your dog to learn it.

How to Train Your Dog to Jump

In the event that your dog has aced fundamental directions, for example, heel, sit and remain, hop would be an exciting order to instruct straightaway. By following the procedure recorded below, you can train your dog to hop.

You will require at any rate one sort of hop to start, for example, the bar. You might need to have a few kinds to mix it up. Set the bars to the most minimal level to ensure that all the dog needs to do first is just a stroll across it.

To start, put a rope on your dog, and hold the chain with two hands. Approach the hop, give the hop order, and lead your pet over the obstacle. When it arrives at the opposite side of the block, give the heel direction. Be liberal with your recognition. As your pet masters the barrier at the most reduced level, continue raising the height at each good result.

The way to teaching the hop order is to have the creature bouncing consistently. If your dog recoils, continue bringing down the level until it, at last, is able to go over it.

If your pet declines to hop all the time, it could be because it has been negated to bounce sometime previously.

When your pet has gotten familiar with the obstacles and will go over them when you give the order, you are ready to let the dog play out the activity all alone with you holding the lead. As it bounces, make sure to have the rope straight before the focal point of the obstacle and afterward bring your arm down like the dog lands.

Give bunches of recognition and treats.

When your dog can heel and bounce without you giving any help, you are presently ready to let the dog play out the lead activity. Approach the obstacle, point to it, and issue the direction to hop.

Rapidly stroll by the block and afterward walk gradually while giving the heel direction and tapping your side.

Be sure not to run when moving toward the obstacle since this energizes dogs and makes them less inclined to follow you. Likewise, continue training fun and praising your pet eagerly. If you feel yourself getting disappointed, stop and accomplish something your pet appreciates more, for example, a round of bringing back an object, so you won't distance it from working with you.

You can utilize the instructions above to train your dog to bounce in a direction.

The first and most significant thing to recall when training a dog is giving it feedback. Continuously reward your dog's good behavior (with a clicker, treat, or a decent stroke) instead of rebuffing adverse action. Remember, dogs need to please; it's a piece of their inherited genetic, so utilize this reality to further your training's success.

It is shrewd to start training your dog from as young as could be allowed. Consequently, in the event that you have a puppy in the house, don't strain yourself unnecessarily to train it during the first few months, otherwise afterward, you will get stressed over the dog's noncompliance.

It is in no way difficult to train a dog, regardless of its age, it's crucial, however, for your dog to recognize you as the pack chief, and you should act in this way from the very first moment.

3 Manners That Your Dog Should Have

- No begging: the most ideal approach to dishearten the continued demand is to guarantee that nobody in the family sneaks nourishment under the table.

The most of human food should not be given to dogs. However, if you have a bit of remaining meat (or something comparable), make your dog hold up until everybody has completed the meal before offering it to it.

- No jumping: if your dog is the friendly sort, they will quickly bounce on outsiders if you allow them to hop on you. Besides, setting the front paws on your shoulders can be a sign of testing your power; so, despite the fact that you may think that it's tender, it should be disheartened.

- Try not to be possessive over toys: For cases when your dog has gotten something it shouldn't or a thing that represents a risk, it is essential that you can remove any object from it. Start by occasionally removing the most loved toys from your dog while it is as yet young.

This may appear to be unfeeling sometimes, yet it just should last for a couple of moments. For example, if it doesn't respond forcefully to you taking back a toy or bone (which will very likely be the situation), offer bunches of recognition and return the thing.

Assuming, nonetheless, there is some snarling or other indication of aggression; it is critical to do the activity for much more of the time and keep the thing for longer timeframes. Your dog should view all toys and bones as yours—you just permit it to play with them.

Obviously, these are only a bunch of things that you should consider when training your dog. If you are experiencing difficulty with training, look for an expert compliance mentor or a veterinarian's counsel.

How to Act Like a Man, Spinning Around, Jump Through Hoops, Roll Over

Do you realize that the most loved trained creature in the global field is a dog?

In a specific part of the world, owning a dog or puppy in a family is viewed as a wellspring of extravagance and a privilege.

Do you have any pet dogs?

How are you investing your energy with it?

Is it accurate to say that you are completing your obligations right now?

If you don't, you should do it.

Your obligation doesn't end by carrying it to your home. An owner is viewed as the best companion of the dog in a living arrangement.

The training is essential since the dogs are known for their unfortunate propensities. Presently, if you neglect to bestow the essential training that will turn it out as an all-around raised dog, it might play with your social nobility, which might be harmed, all things considered, before anything else.

The best way of training is to be consistent, especially if the dog is at the incipient stage or a young puppy.

Is it accurate to say that you can have a puppy?

In the event that it is, you should begin training it once it arrives at the age of 6 to 8 months. The puppy stays like aboard at this stage, and you can compose whatever you like on it.

Always remember, if the seeds of compliance are planted inside it now, it will prove to be fruitful all through life.

By what method would it be advisable for you to start the instructing of compliances? From the earliest moment, attempt to build up the connection between both of you. The liking must be based on respect and not like between companions. Dogs, being wild creatures, like to live in packs, and every one of these packs stays heavily influenced by an alpha dog.

This alpha dog has an unconquerable force, and this makes different dogs bow before it. So, if you show your dog your strength, you will be the pioneer of the pack from the very start.

The following part is the direction training. Each direction must be unambiguous, explicit, and must comprise of a single word. This empowers the dog to grasp the rules effectively and act from the perspective of that.

The utilization of the "No" direction must be made carefully since this word happens to be generally helpful in the jargon of either a dog or man. At whatever point, it does anything, and if you don't care for that, you should state "No" completely.

The puppy won't get your language; however, being savvy will show off your outward appearance and non-verbal communication. This will empower you to train it and also to apply your control. Obviously, you should incorporate the training too. This is important and supports the dog to catch on quickly.

Dogs are the most well-known trained creatures as they are considered man's closest companions. Notwithstanding, this isn't always the real situation.

Your dog may likewise wreck your life if it isn't appropriately trained.

It is essential to show your dog to carry on particularly openly. If your dog is very much trained, you are sure to carry your dog with you anywhere you need it.

In the event that you are unable to the direction of your dog to carry on or have it plunk down, it might humiliate you from others.

What's more, far more terrible, it may bark and seize individuals making them be terrified. If these sorts of circumstances are annoying you, at that point, the time has come to change the behavior of your dog.

Dogs can be compared to small kids. They should be shown some correct habits and how to carry on particularly with others. Much the same as kids, you need to enable your dog to build up its social viewpoint and act appropriately.

Train your dog to turn into a social being.

In the event that you make some hard memories training your dog, you can carry it to an expert coach. Obviously, this will mean you need to spend some money.

If you are on a limited spending plan and are not ready to contract a coach, you don't have a choice but to train your dog yourself.

If you don't have the foggiest idea of how to do it, you can get a few books and articles on the best way to show your dog how to act. A few materials offer a total bit-by-bit technique on showing your dog to follow directions that you will give.

Remember that you need a great deal of tolerance in teaching your dog as you have to rehash again-and-again the things that you need to impart in it.

Giving it a prize is additionally a smart thought for it to understand that it is progressing admirably.

It might be a dreary errand, yet it is all worthy, despite all the trouble. If you can show your dog how to act appropriately and cause it to follow directions, both of you will be placated and cheerful.

Teach Your Dog to Spin Around

Turning is a simple trick to show to your dog. First, stand out enough to be noticed, utilizing a treat. Grasping the treat, hold it over its nose, and gradually move it in an enormous hover simply over its head.

It ought to follow your hand. Keep moving your handful-circle and, if your dog follows your hand to finish the circle, acclaim and give it the treat. Rehash those steps a couple of times, permitting it to become accustomed to the movements.

When it is finally reliably following your handful-circle, include the verbal prompt "Spin Around."

After it is good at finishing one full turn, you can include more circles before giving it the treat. At that point, you can begin requesting 2 to 3 twists—or significantly more—before you give it the treat. After a couple of effective repetitions, utilize your hand movement without the treat, so your dog doesn't get reliant on doing the trick, dependent on whether it sees an obvious threat or not.

Keep in mind, keep training sessions short and consistently!

Jumping Through Hoops

While teaching this trick, it is significant not to hold the loop at a level that will make it too hard for your dog to bounce through. Get hold of a circle, take a treat in your other hand and at the opposite side of the loop. Make sure that your dog can see the treat.

The point here is to get your dog to pass through the circle instead of going around it to get the treat. If your dog circumvents the loop instead of passing through it, don't compensate it with the treat. When your dog experiences the circle, it gives the direction 'ruckus'. As we did in the past tricks, rehash this procedure for 10 or 15 minutes.

This is somewhat more troublesome than the past tricks, and to make it simpler, you can begin with the circle laying on the ground before raising the height. Rehash this trick for a couple of different sessions, and your dog will, in the end, get it right.

Teach a Dog to Roll Over

Rollover is a charming trick that is simple and enjoyable to show your dog. It is useful if your dog knows the "down" order before you begin showing this trick.

- Ask your dog to play out a "down" position before you.
- Kneel adjacent to your dog and hold a little, yummy treat to the side of its head close to its nose.
- Move your hand from its nose toward its shoulder, attracting it to move level on its side.
- Try this a couple of times, acclaim, and treat each time it follows the treat and lies level on its side with its head on the floor.
- Now proceed with the further movement of your hand, holding a treat, when it is lying level, from its shoulder to its spine. This should make it roll onto its back.
- Continue moving the treat hand, so it rolls onto the opposite side.
- When it is reliably following the treat right around in a "turn over", include the verbal prompt "Roll Over."

- Gradually diminish the hand movement and treat bait until your dog can play out the trick on only a verbal prompt.

Mark the Spot, Shake It Off

Your dog can be trained to go to an imprint, which may be an X set apart on the floor with tape, a spot board, a bit of cardboard, a bit of fabric, or a tangle or bed.

These imprints can be utilized at a particular area in your home to give a spot to your dog to go when you have to control undesirable conduct or can be utilized in a wide range of situations. For example, if you have to take your dog out in broad daylight or to work, to guide your dog to a fitting spot where it is sheltered and not causing an issue, etc.

Dogs that are involved in showbiz are frequently trained to go to an imprint so they are in a suitable spot for recording or playing out a trick. To show your dog to go to an imprint, you need to show your dog to focus on a specific thing, for example, an X, and go to that spot and pause there.

Is essential that you will instruct your dog to commands like "Down/Stay" or "Sit/Stay" preceding instructing it to go to an imprint, with the goal that when your dog focuses on its imprint, it recognizes what practices to perform there.

These lessons require a tad of bearing and training to get your dog to comprehend and perform; notwithstanding, even young dogs can learn how to go to an imprint. When working with a young dog, you should continue instructional meetings properly and don't require the dog to remain excessively long at the imprint. A young dog has a limited ability to focus, and setting unreasonable goals will only cause disappointment.

It would help if you decided in advance what your dog's imprint will be. In the event that the behavior you want to teach is something that you need your dog to act in an assortment of spots, you will require something versatile. You may utilize a dog bed as an imprint at home, or a little tangle could be utilized at home and taken with you out and about. Showbiz dogs frequently use an X made with paint or veiling tape on the floor as an imprint.

You can use anything, even a cloth or facecloth, to make an imprint, as long as you will always use the same once decided.

After founding an imprint, then decide what action you need your dog to perform at its imprint before training it. Do you maybe need it to plunk down or rest?

As we said, you will need to encourage your dog to sit and sit down before instructing to go to its imprint, so you don't overload it. Concoct a verbal order, for example, 'tangle', 'spot', or 'imprint', which you will use to guide your dog to its imprint.

You will require a lot of treats and possibly a clicker to reward your dog's behavior during training. A few coaches also utilize a training stick to guide their dog to the imprint. This is particularly helpful if the area of their imprint is going to move, for example, for exhibitions.

Shake It Off

Have you at any point had a wet dog on your hands (after a shower or a stroll outside in the downpour) and just wished it would "shake" its coat.

On the other hand, shouldn't something be said about when your dog moves on the ground and gathers bits of leaves, grass, and who-knows-what-else in its coat?

If solitary, it would take off quite a bit of that dirt and bits with a decent "shake" first. At that point, you'd be much happier thinking of it hopping in the vehicle or going into the house, isn't that so?

To get our dogs to "shake" on command, we began the training in the bath. Our main goal is just not to let them escape the tub UNTIL they shook. Generally, each dog would want to "shake" in any event twice during their shower—all alone.

So that gave us multiple times to adulate them for performing such conduct—without us requesting it!

After that, you just have to introduce the verbal command "shake" every time the conduct is carried out until you get obedience to the order.

Chapter 8.
THE SECRETS OF LIVING IN HARMONY WITH YOUR DOG

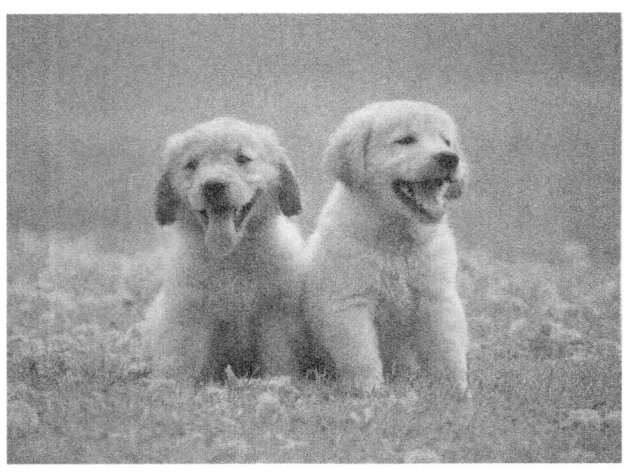

10 Most Significant Guidelines If You Need to Live in Harmony with Your Dog

1. Accept that They're Only Dogs

He/she is a dog and will carry on like a dog, similar to their temperament. You can cherish your dog like your youngster, and there aren't any issues with that.

In any case, understand that dogs some of the time bark, dig into the ground, bite on things, and occasionally get filthy. Practices like these are regular and not an issue.

If they exaggerate some of them, at that point, we can discuss awful or undesirable behavior. However, after all that, it can merely be a type of disappointment on their part, or absence of activity and not a genuine social issue.

2. Speak in Dog Language

This might be the hardest piece of all.

"I love my dog like my own kid" and "It understands what I say to it."

My god, how frequently did I advise that to myself or heard it from other dog owners?

I needed to understand that dogs don't comprehend human language. I originally thought it could be possible my dog would even communicate in 3 distinct dialects (I lived with it in 3 unique nations).

But it was not so. Dogs get the mood, tone, and sound, yet not words or sentences. They have their own particular manner of conveying, which isn't as muddled as our own.

Consequently, I strongly suggest learning somewhat more of their 'language' than expecting them to get familiar with our own.

3. Find Your Own Dog's Character

Numerous individuals believe that a few breeds are dangerous, while some are sweet or savvy. I will disclose to you a mystery: each dog has an alternate personality. I had three dogs of a similar breed, yet every one of them had their own attitude.

Obviously, they had comparative characters (they were all so adorable). However, each had its own little peculiarities that made the entire excursion together progressively wonderful.

If you have one dog of a specific breed and you decide to purchase another relative of a similar breed: please don't expect that they will absolutely act similarly on the grounds that they won't.

I truly don't need any dog owner to be disillusioned. I have met a pit bull that was a blessed angel and a Chihuahua that was a little fiend. They all have their own personalities.

4. Be a Leader

Dogs usually live in a gathering, or all the more precisely, a pack. Their family is their pack. They use non-verbal communication of different individuals from the 'pack' to realize what their position is. They likewise utilize their own non-verbal communication toward another part to impart or show them their position.

If you need to be the person who sets the guidelines, at that point, you should be the more grounded and progressively prevailing one. Be confident and know precisely what you need, and your dog will tail it.

Trust me; it's harder to accomplish than it sounds. You should not be forceful or destructive, yet you must be certain about yourself. In the event that you dither, your dog will be the chief, and it will tell you what you have to manage.

Positive Reinforcement

An ideal approach to encourage helpful tricks or excellent behavior is to fortify your dog's actions at the perfect time. This doesn't imply that you generally need to stroll around your home with a sack of bacon or chicken so that every time your dog accomplishes something great, you put a treat in their mouth. Not in the slightest degree.

You need to comprehend that the best support from you is your consideration. Envision your dog like a 3-year-old kid who shouts, yells, and cries until one of the parents at long last asks he/her, "What is the issue?."

Dogs likewise need consideration; thusly your touch or a game time can be utilized as uplifting feedback, rather than a bit of bacon.

6. Comprehend the Vitality Level of Your Dog and Your Own Also

I have seen so often dog owners battle with their dogs, not on the grounds that they didn't adore them, but since they were not a decent match.

Are you not catching my meaning?

When your way of life is about recreation, or maybe you are simply not a functioning individual, however, you get a dog with a high vitality level, with a very dynamic nature—trust me; your life will be a horrendous experience soon. This isn't on the grounds that you are an awful individual or potentially your dog is awful, but since your needs are entirely different.

Most behavior issues originate from the absence of activity. When I was 4 years of age, we had a hyperactive cocker spaniel, which my parents needed to offer a way to a nearby family companion, as my mum couldn't cope with staying aware of two little children with a hyperactive dog.

Our companion instead had two adolescent young men who cherished climbing. They took the dog all over the place, so they never had any behavior issues with the dog, as it had the option to live as indicated by its tendency.

For an extremely longtime span, I thought my folks parted with it since it was me the one unable to handle it appropriately. I rebuffed myself for that, and I concluded that I needed to get the hang of everything about dogs.

In any event, when I read many books about dogs and their breeds, I required time to perceive that despite the fact that it was difficult and frightful for me, it was really the best for it.

I don't mean that you need to part from it in the event that you have a hyperactive dog. Perhaps the dog could be a major part of your life to show you something. If you constantly needed to climb, take up cycling, running, and so forth, at that point, possibly you picked this dog to begin another lifestyle... You never know!

Suppose you find that isn't the situation. In that case, you, despite everything, have the other extraordinary alternative to hiring a dog walker who can exercise your dog for you and drain its energy.

7. Harmony with All Relatives

Attempt to speak with your whole family, so every part practices similar guidelines with the dog. If the mum doesn't want the dog going up to the dinner table, however, the youngster gives it a huge bit of meat next to the table; at that point, you have to have a serious family meeting and set down all the standards.

Rules will make you and your family's life simpler. Clear principles and limits will make it simpler for your dog to follow.

8. Understand Your Dog's Changing Behavior

So frequently, I meet individuals who complain about their dogs eating their couches and shoes.

At that point, I ask them: "What might you do if you were shut in a jail cell consistently for the majority of the day? Would you be disappointed?" obviously, the appropriate response is 'yes'. At this point, contemplate your dog's day-by-day schedule.

Suppose it's truly frustrating; at that point attempt some toys to try animating its mind. Remember that a dog can likewise be worn out by something. However, there are such a significant number of places these days where you can purchase intriguing new toys for your pet.

9. The Old Dog Can Become Familiar with Another Trick

Training and teaching are the best exercises for any dog, especially when its temper is terrible. Teaching your dog to do new exercise isn't just valuable to show up with your loved ones, yet also essential to keep your dog occupied and tired.

10. Exercise

Perhaps this ought to be the principal point on this rundown. Any sort of terrible behavior can be significantly diminished with customary exercise. Dogs usually are able to go across 10km every day. Along these lines, if we wall them in our home or nursery alone, it's not shocking if they are then baffled and bark, bite and bounce.

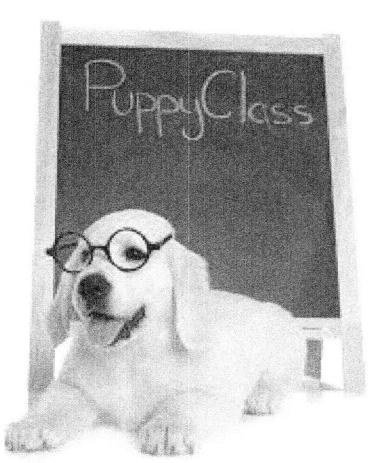

They can get forceful from the absence of activity. For this reason, before you give your dog a harsh judgment, it would be ideal if you consider how frequently you take it out, how regularly it has the chance to run like there's no tomorrow. Before you abandon your "crazy dog", you should help it to exercise consistently, and you will be astounded at the adjustment in its behavior just as you like.

Worst Puppy Training Mistakes

- Train your dog for a really long time. Long instructional courses are not effective enough for a few reasons. Your dog may get exhausted (particularly a puppy or young with a limited ability to focus!), or you may begin getting drained and not focus on what your dog is doing. What's more, truly, it's a great deal for your dog to take all in! Can you recall those long hours of school classes that killed your mind when you were young? An instructional dog course does exactly the same as your dog's brain. For this reason, shorter is better— think about just 10 minutes of training or something like that.

- Beating a dead... Well, you know the idiom. Regularly when a dog misunderstands something, individuals simply continue having them do it again-and-again, maybe believing that by doing so, the dog will "lurch" upon the right reaction. Nonetheless, if your dog misses the point on multiple occasions in succession—STOP. This implies you are not giving your dog enough data. In the event that you continue doing it, your dog is simply going to get baffled and quit attempting, and you will become irritated.

- Training when not in the right mood—this is a catastrophe waiting to happen. Your dog commits an error, and abruptly, you are venting out your dissatisfaction, outrage, and so on it. Instead, hang out and cuddle with it on the sofa until your disposition improves, or simply calm yourself doing something else you like even without your dog.

- Mixing rewarding and rectifying feedback techniques has been deductively demonstrated that uplifting feedback strategies produce preferred outcomes over rectification-based training. By far worse, nonetheless, is blending the two. It creates a mistaking climate for the dog, which can't be sure whether it will be rebuffed or compensated. This causes the dog's inability to do what he is asked to do—would you hazard offering something if you didn't know whether you would have been compensated or rebuffed?

- Abusing the clicker—there are rules to utilizing the clicker accurately. Normal errors incorporate clicking and not compensating your dog (once is fine, however, if you continue doing it, that clicker will lose its incentive to the dog) and clicking more than once per behavior (dogs move quick and in the event that you click several times for one conduct, your dog has no clue what you were looking for).

- Not enough practice. This botch is a big deal since it will influence your dog's presentation. Numerous individuals take a dog compliance class, and during that time, they practice with their dogs. They learn the practices, and everything goes well. Easily a couple of months forward, or a year even, the owners will be disappointed on the grounds that their dog won't sit to welcome, etc.... This is because their dog hasn't been approached to do any practice on it since the class. Dogs' aptitudes get corroded, simply like it happen for us—would you be able to tackle an arithmetical exercise in the event that somebody exhibited it to you once and then you never practice it again? Most likely not, except if you use them in your day-by-day life. Along these lines, make sure to keep up on your dog's abilities—remember only a few minutes daily is everything that is necessary.

• Command bothering: this is a major mistake that most dog owners make—rehashing prompts. You state "sit", your dog doesn't react, and you say "sit" once more. Furthermore, once more. At that point, you wonder why your dog doesn't respond to the first attempt when you give an order. All things considered, when you are training your dog, you don't have to repeat the order a second or even fourth time. Instead, in this way, you have now instructed it that the signal is "Sit, sit, sit, sit." And your dog will rely on that fourth prompt before reacting next time. Instead, just state it once. If your dog doesn't come, go get it. If it still doesn't work, there must be a reason why your dog is not responding. So you will need to investigate and don't give the order again until it's sorted.

• Training always in a similar spot— if you have a dog that obeys on consummately at home while is then uncontrollable anywhere else, you are blameworthy of this slip-up. Dogs don't sum up—which means if you show your dog to sit in your parlor and, at that point, request that it sit upstairs or outside, it may not do it. To have a respectful dog all over the place, make certain to take your training out-and-about and practice in lots of different spots.

• Too many treats—while treats are, for most dogs, an incredible method to begin the training procedure, remember to include acclaim, toys, and "genuine prizes" like petting and play when your dog learns tricks. Otherwise, you will have one of those dogs that possibly work if you have nourishment on you.

Dog Treating

Treats and bites should just make up 10% of a dog's daily calories. To get a better thought of what number of treats that is, ask your vet. They can make a suggestion based on the treats your dog loves, its weight, and how dynamic it is.

Obviously, dogs love treats, and they will not refuse them even if not needed.

What're more, individuals love giving their dogs treats. It's a method to bond with your pet, and that is something to be thankful for. So you can simply give them each in turn.

Try Veggies and Fruit

You can avoid the locally acquired tidbits that are high in fat, sugar, and frequent additives, and you can try to offer your dog a few vegetables. "Give them a baby carrot, a green bean, some broccoli". Those have practically no calories, and dogs may not care at all in case you're not giving them something substantial and greasy. They simply need you to provide them with something.

Dogs are prepared to eat all nourishments, possibly. Therefore, vegetables can be an excellent nibble choice for your dog. You can attempt some fruit as well—banana cuts, berries, watermelon, and apple cuts (without any seeds, obviously).

On the contrary, you should avoid grapes, raisins, onions, chocolate, and anything with caffeine, as those can be poisonous to dogs.

Dog Nutrition

Maybe the most well-known inquiry pet owners pose to their veterinarian is, "What should I feed my dog with?"

When feeding your dog, you need a well-adjusted eating routine that is focused on its general wellbeing and prosperity. To see how and with what to sustain your dog, you have to understand what the wholesome prerequisites of dogs are and how these necessities have developed through the procedure of natural growth.

As a species, the dog belongs to the world of carnivores, a huge group of mammalian creatures with an elaborate tooth structure.

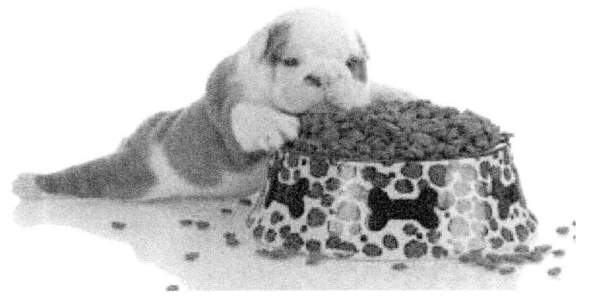

The dietary needs of creatures having a place in this mammal's category are different. A few members from this species have a complete necessity for meat in their eating routine (called committed or genuine carnivores); while others can meet their prerequisites through eating plant material (herbivores) or a blend of meat and plants (omnivores). Cat is a case of a committed meat-eater, dairy animals are a case of herbivores, and humans and dogs are two instances of omnivores.

In light of dogs' dietary needs, both their tooth structure and intestinal tract have gotten adjusted to an omnivorous eating routine. This implies that dogs can meet their nourishing needs under typical conditions by eating a blend of plants and meet nourishments.

What Are the Healthful Necessities for Dogs?

The six fundamental supplements are water, proteins, fats, sugars, minerals, and nutrients. These essential supplements are required as a component of the dog's ordinary eating regimen and are engaged with the entirety of the body's fundamental necessity.

There are also some supplements made with all the nutrients needed. However, even if the average measures of certain supplements are known, they sometimes have been identified as poisoning consequences.

Dietary rules have been created by the Association of American Feed Control Officials (AAFCO). AAFCO rules are the general guidelines for the nourishing substance needed for pet feeding. Ensure that your dog's nourishment fulfills the AAFCO guidelines.

Remember that these are very important rules to follow, and your dog requires relying upon them for its well-being status. Address your veterinarian for more data on explicit supplements that your specific dog may require.

What Should I Look for in Dog Food?

The best counsel you can get about feeding your dog is this: feed your dog the most excellent nourishment you can manage.

The contrasts between top-notch nutrition and cheaper food are not found on the sustenance mark; they are found in the quality and wellspring of nutrients. Two dog nourishments may each contain 27% protein; however, they may be immeasurably unique with regards to edibility.

Pet nourishment supplements are recorded by request of weight. Every nutrient is weighed when added to the cluster of nourishment, and some ingredients, such as crisp meat, contain a great deal of water, quite a bit of which is lost during handling. This implies a dry eating routine that highlights corn as the main ingredient, which is healthfully better than one based on the meat first.

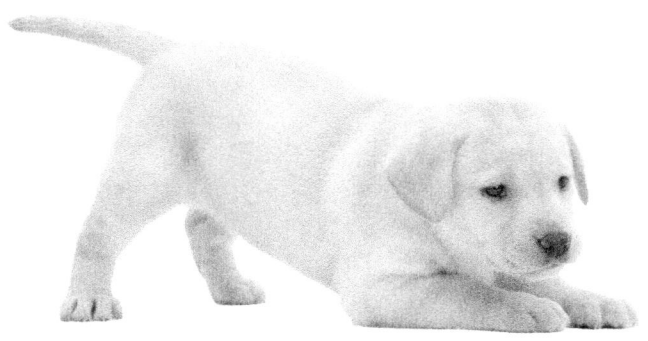

Training your puppy is essentially forming this specific thought into your puppy dog—it isn't the big cheese inside the household family. And you, as the puppy pet owner, should set yourself up just like the big enchilada in the pack.

Inside the puppy's thinking manner, this furnishes you with the legitimate right to impact the puppy's propensities and the directions that the puppy must follow.

Start the way toward this methodology by looking legitimately at the puppy eye-to-eye until, in the long run, the puppy turns or looks away. These are extensive lead-dog dealings of which the puppy dog will positively usually have a comprehension of.

Potty training is among the most critical types of activity expected for a new puppy dog. As we said, you can potty train your puppy dog basically by getting it out in the open each time you assume the puppy will need to discard "something" every single time the puppy disposes of itself outside the house. You should just reward the puppy pleasantly by utilizing doggie snacks or verbal commendations.

Social training is one more fundamental activity. Teach your own puppy dog to be amiable alongside different pets or with individuals by allowing the puppy to be close to many unfamiliar individuals.

Staying near unknown individuals alongside local pets, for example, in a dog park, will indeed teach your puppy never to begin barking at everyone it spots and never to get unfriendly to different dogs.

Getting acquainted with unfamiliar individuals, just as different pets, is a significant piece for transforming your dog into a beautiful family pet that won't become brutal against someone with no explanation.

Also, make sure to mentor your puppy in some crucial directions. The specific trends like come, remain, and sit are commonly trained basically by ordering the particular conduct verbally, causing the puppy to do it physically, and finally rewarding it once done. These sorts of directions are of help in a wide range of conditions, so attempt to instruct your puppy concerning these sets of commands as soon as possible.

There are plenty of books on this subject on the market, so thanks again for choosing this one!

Every effort was made to ensure that it is full of as much useful information as possible, please enjoy it!

Finally, if you found this book useful in any way, a review on Amazon is always appreciated!

Printed in Great Britain
by Amazon

61912194R00092